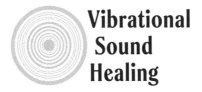

Vibrational Sound Healing

....

"A clear, comprehensive study of the miracle of sound. Well researched and easy to read and to experience directly."

TIM WHEATER, AWARD-WINNING COMPOSER,
FLAUTIST, VOCALIST, PERFORMER, AND PUBLIC SPEAKER

"Erica fills in the gaps in our understanding of how sound can heal and change us. Plain and easy to understand, it's a pleasure to read."

MARK SWAN, GONG MASTER

"Like the resonance of ancient Sona given as a gift from the Divine, indented into the stone walls of great temples by the voices of the priests and priestesses, Erica has crafted a fascinating sculpture of sound in *Vibrational Sound Healing*. May this sonic healing resonate deep within our souls forever!"

STEWART PEARCE, MASTER OF VOICE
AND SOUND ALCHEMIST

Vibrational Sound Healing

Take Your Sonic Vitamins
with Tuning Forks, Singing Bowls,
Chakra Chants, Angelic Vibrations,
and Other Sound Therapies

ERICA LONGDON

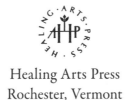

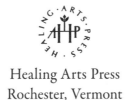

Healing Arts Press
Rochester, Vermont

Healing Arts Press
One Park Street
Rochester, Vermont 05767
www.HealingArtsPress.com

Healing Arts Press is a division of Inner Traditions International

*Note to the reader: This book is intended as an informational guide. The remedies,
approaches, and techniques described herein are meant to supplement, and not to be a
substitute for, professional medical care or treatment. They should not be used to treat a
serious ailment without prior consultation with a qualified health care professional.*

Cataloging-in-Publication Data for this title is available from the Library of Congress

ISBN 978-1-64411-161-1 (print)
ISBN 978-1-64411-162-8 (ebook)

Printed and bound in the United States by Versa Press, Inc.

10   9   8   7   6   5   4   3   2

Text design and layout by Virginia Scott Bowman
This book was typeset in Garamond Premier Pro with Spirits Soft used as the display
typeface

To send correspondence to the author of this book, mail a first-class letter to the author
c/o Inner Traditions • Bear & Company, One Park Street, Rochester, VT 05767, and
we will forward the communication, or contact the author directly at **angelhandsheal
.co.uk**.

◆ ◆ ◆

The universe

doesn't use

language.

It speaks

vibration.

Contents

Sonic Vitamins for Sound Health

My Journey into Sound Health

BEFORE I LAUNCH INTO THE MAIN BODY of this book, it may be helpful to know about my journey; I was a nonbeliever before I became a psychic, therapist, and healer. When I have chosen to study or learn from someone, I have always found it helpful to know their credentials. Maybe that's because I am a Libra; we love the mystical yet are notorious for wanting to know the facts. Perhaps you do too.

As a child, I had always felt that I didn't quite "fit the mold." I was told to be a good girl and not challenge what my elders and superiors told me was acceptable behavior. I was expected to work hard, get good exam results, and head to university. Thus qualified, I would get a good job where I could meet a suitable man in order to settle down to secure family life (believe me, that was the 1950s wisdom instilled into all grammar school girls). The thought made me shudder. I was a wild-spirited tomboy who loved running free in nature and climbing to the tips of thirty-foot beech trees to cling onto their flimsy crowns swaying in the wind. Two things occur to me about this: first, it is a miracle that I am here to write these words, and second, my mother would have a fit if she'd known what I had been doing.

Nevertheless, I conformed to the system until I escaped uniform suburbia for London where I landed my first job in television. Yet despite a wonderful career traveling the world and working with astoundingly creative people, I felt a void. Externally, I seemed to live a glamourous life, but nobody saw the lost little girl who quivered inside and felt that she was never good enough. My belief systems were completely secular, so in my psyche, there was no one to turn to for advice. Something wasn't right, and I knew it. I needed a wake-up call. But if someone had told me then that I would talk to angels and work as a psychic, I would have laughed out loud.

My wake-up call came in 1988 as I was driving through London's morning rush hour traffic on the way to a long shift as a television voice-over. I was crossing a busy junction when I was broadsided at speed, and as my car arced through the air, I clearly remember turning my head to look through the passenger window and seeing the sky and clouds. Just as I'd seen in films, everything moved in slow motion, and I thought to myself: *Is this it? Am I going to die?* But I felt no fear, and it was as if I were in a bubble. I have no recollection of the final impact with the ground. The car landed on the driver's side, and I lay, still strapped in my seat, covered in glass from the shattered windows.

I checked that all my limbs seemed to be free and working and stood up, my head poking through the passenger window. Broken glass poured off me like water, yet I suffered not a single scratch.

It didn't occur to me in the shock of that moment that I was being watched over, that I had a purpose in my life for which I was being preserved. I know that now. Something else I didn't know was that, having been told by a gynecological consultant I would never be able to have children, I was pregnant.

As wake-up calls go, this one was massive, but still I continued to play my role in what I had been told was normal life and juggled being a working woman, wife, and mother. There was no time for reflection and self-knowledge. So, because I hadn't heeded the first wake-up call, life gave me a second slap upside the head. As a result of the car accident, I suffered latent trauma two years later when my back locked and caused me incredible pain. I couldn't move! This time I had to stop and listen.

I had a deep intuitive knowing that mainstream pharmacological and surgical medicine didn't hold the answer. I discovered cranial osteopathy and from there I was on the road to complementary therapies. As I began to heal my body, I became aware of how much I needed to heal my mind, heart, and soul. For the first time, I was *aware* and *listening,* two primary lessons I needed to learn to work with sound. I studied to become a masseuse and then a Reiki master. Once I felt the Reiki energy running through my hands, I knew that I had no interest in resuming "normal life." I was heading toward the person I was always meant to be. My journey led me to meet some beautiful and wise healers. It didn't matter that I had taken forty years to find this path; my wrong turns simply served to deliver perspective, so the lessons were never wasted.

When we choose change, people expand with us, or our paths diverge. The pace of my awakening increased, and the third major shift occurred: my divorce. To the outside world it looked like a catastrophe. To me it felt like being released from the prison of a life where I didn't belong and hadn't known how to escape. I flowed into a new beginning and expanded life using exercise, sound bathing, and energetic vibration. I allowed change and synchronicity to guide me, and above all, I trusted the universe, that all-encompassing vibratory plane of existence that guides us to our unique and authentic life if only we will tune in and listen. Being prepared to stop and listen is the first step toward sound health. Was it easy? Certainly not! Growth rarely is. However, the alternative of the status quo would have been disastrous.

When we listen, the truth can be revealed to us. To discover who I am was a major journey that grew from my awakening. I found myself surrounded by world-class mediums, and although I studied mediumship at the famous Arthur Findlay College, I knew, deep down, that was not who I am. I have spent time in shamanic and Wiccan circles and ceremonies, both of which expanded my connection to our Mother Earth. Yet I was not home. I found my tribe among angel intuitives and complementary healing practitioners as a healer who is psychic. Never be afraid to search until you find your fit. I hold qualifications in oral communication, advanced massage technique, ear candling, stress counseling, psychology, meditation, and sound healing. I am a Reiki master and angel intuitive, and I play the flute. Yet when I am working with a client, I cannot and do not subdivide my treatments by those delineations. I am a healer; I listen to my clients and bring forth whatever they need that day. It is a case of being in tune.

 When you find your own note, your place in the symphony of life, you will come into holistic resonance and become your own healer. Why? Because everything is vibration. When you find harmony, you allow sound health.

Although I have studied the use and application of sound for therapeutic healing using many of the disciplines discussed in this book, my own journey has taken me to specialize in using tuning forks. To work with sound healing, as in the medical field, a broad grounding and knowledge of all the systems involved is essential, but ultimately most physicians make a choice. They may choose general practice, or they may choose to specialize in endocrinology, gastroenterology, or one of the myriad branches of medicine. Similarly, my initial studies encompassed a broad spectrum of sound healing modalities. I have since chosen to focus on working with tuning forks—it's my thing.

As you read about the sonic vitamins in this book, you may find yourself particularly drawn to one more than another. Or you may try some of them and find that some work better for you than others. The same is true of allopathic medicine. Some drugs work better than others for some patients. It is the responsibility of each of us to listen to our body and work with the system that brings about a better quality of life or healing.

Vibration, the Foundation of Sound Healing

UNDERSTANDING VIBRATION

If you want to find the secrets of the universe, think in terms of energy, frequency and vibration.

SCIENTIST NIKOLA TESLA, WHOSE WORK
WAS SO FAR AHEAD OF HIS TIME THAT
HE WAS RIDICULED AND SHUNNED

Vibration comes in many forms. It is felt when an earthquake shakes a building; it is seen when a high note shatters a glass; it is heard as frequencies carried over air, which our ears perceive as sound, speech, and music; or it is our thoughts as they create electrical and vibrational impulses. Vibration is the foundation of sound and the carrier of sonic vitamins.

The study of vibration and the use of it to improve our lives is becoming more common. Damien Coyle, professor of neurotechnology, is developing neurotechnology for the physically impaired that "measures and translates brainwaves into control signals" for communication.[1] At MIT, the Massachusetts Institute of Technology, a device that utilizes subvocalization is now in use. Subvocalization is the practice of silently saying words in your head. It's common when we read but it has only recently begun to be used as a way to interact with computers and mobile devices. To that end, MIT researchers have created a device worn on the face that can measure neuromuscular signals triggered when you subvocalize. These signals can then be interpreted and used to instruct computers and mobile devices.[2]

Japanese author and researcher Masaru Emoto recorded his remarkable findings of the effects of human consciousness, thought, intention, and the spoken word and music on the molecular structure of water in his book *The Hidden Messages in Water*.

Vibration is everywhere, even in space; it is matter, and it matters! Consider that we can't see a phone signal or the impulse that attracts two magnetic forces. They are there, nevertheless. But if vibration is not usually visible, how have we come to understand it? One way is through the science of cymatics, from the Greek word *kyma* meaning "wave," which is the process of making vibration visible. The term was coined by Hans Jenny, a Swiss scientist and accomplished pianist who taught at the Rudolph Steiner School in Zurich before taking up a career in medicine. In the study of cymatics, vibration causes the oscillation of particles or water to form patterns on a membrane (see Vitamin C).

Life is a macrocosm and a microcosm simultaneously. If vibration is found in the vastness of space and in the material formation of objects on Earth, it is also found in the organs and cells of the human body where vibration occurs naturally in every moment, even though we cannot see it. Scientists have documented a conversation between the heart and the brain, both electrical and magnetic, in which the heart is by far the dominant transmitter. Its transmissions are 5,000 times stronger than those of the brain. When we feel something strongly, the electrical impulse we create has the power to change us. That is how (and why) affirmations work. The optimum electrical frequency to harmonize your heart and brain is a very low frequency, the same frequency that whales use to communicate, at 0.1 Hz, just on the threshold of feeling and hearing.* Buddhist monks are so adept at tuning in to this conversation that they can use their heart to send messages to their brain to alter and control the body's state, including its heart rate, temperature, and so on. When they are meditating, they are not always in the ultraslow brain wave state of delta rhythm. They can create a gamma brain wave, which is faster than the beta rhythm associated with normal waking consciousness and can be used to change bodily conditions.

 The heart working in concert with the brain—the heart's intention—is like a magic wand, so be careful where you point it!

If vibration is all around us, in what other ways does it influence our lives? The Schumann Frequency, also known as the Schumann Resonance of our home, planet Earth, is measured in Hertz, and there is solid scientific evidence to point to its existence. Civil engineer Trevor English explains, "that there is a great deal of electrical activity between the surface of the Earth and the ionosphere. Some of this is in the form of standing waves of electricity. These standing waves are

---

*Sound frequencies are measured in Hertz (Hz) or cycles per second (CPS). The way these are measured is identical; it is just the nomenclature that is different. In your journey ahead in this book, Hz is used as the frame of reference.

known as Schumann Resonances."[3] Electromagnetic waves generated and excited by lightning discharges in the cavity formed between the Earth's surface and the ionosphere become trapped. Sometimes these waves come into resonance to become part of the Schumann Resonance, Earth's heartbeat, which occurs in the extremely low frequency (ELF) portion of Earth's electromagnetic field spectrum.[4]

In other words, the Schumann Resonance creates the vibrational soup in which we exist. We cannot separate ourselves from it. When astronauts leave Earth, there are consequences for their health. The Schumann Resonances help maintain natural human rhythms such as hormone production, melatonin levels, menstruation, and sleep cycles. The astronauts felt unwell and were unable to sleep when deprived of this vital frequency, so NASA installed the Schumann simulator to mimic the Earth's frequency.[5] You may experience the same symptoms as the astronauts did in space if the Schumann Frequency around you is disrupted by metal wiring, metal roofs, and reinforced concrete. This might explain why industrial and high-rise buildings filled with computer equipment and electronic devices are sometimes said to have "sick building syndrome." People have headaches, become irritable, and feel drained as their natural biorhythms entrain to the frequency of the building instead of the Earth. On Earth, we are constantly affected by the Schumann Resonance, and our thoughts and emotional state (and thus our vibrational state) interact with and affect it in turn. "The similarity of the 7.8-Hertz Earth resonance and human brainwave rhythms was quickly identified after the Schumann resonances were first measured, and early studies were able to demonstrate a correlation between these resonances and brain rhythms."[6]

Have you ever felt that time seems to be quickening? Scientific research shows that this may be true.

For many years, the Schumann Resonance's frequency has hovered at a steady 7.83 Hz with only slight variations. In June 2014, that apparently changed. Monitors at the Russian Space Observing System showed a sudden spike in activity to around 8.5 Hz. Since then, they have recorded days where the Schumann was as high as 16.5 Hz. At first, they thought their equipment was malfunctioning but later learned the data was accurate.[7]

Is the Earth's frequency speeding up? As we age, that is a common perception as we feel we are "running out of time," but this phenomenon has been experienced by people of all ages. Since the Schumann Frequency is said to be in tune with the human brain's alpha and theta states, acceleration of the Schumann Frequency may be why it often feels like time has sped up and events and changes in our life are happening more rapidly.

As the Schumann Resonance has been seen to spike, it is reasonable to assume that this could cause a parallel reaction in the human brain. Some commentators have expounded that our response to an increase in brain frequency is a sense of heightened consciousness or awakening, as new age parlance would express it. In neurofeedback terminology, progressing from 7.83 Hz, a relaxed or dreamy state of mind, to anything between 12 to 15 Hz would take our state of mind to a higher alpha state, which could be described as "awakened calm." In this state, our thought processes are clear and focused, yet we are balanced and calm. This has been expressed as being "in the zone" or "going with the flow." It is a very creative place to be.

However, all change and adjustment has its side effects. Just as a computer needs to shut down and reboot, so our system requires rest to assimilate this new state of being. Some people may find they are tired, drained, dizzy, or have mood swings. Sometimes we simply feel strange without being able to put a finger on why. However, understanding that you are undergoing a recalibration can make the process less unsettling. It helps to remember that it is all part of your awakening to keep pace with the ascension of our planetary home to a higher rate of vibration, or dimension, and thus a more compassionate plane of existence.

As Mr. Spock might have raised an eyebrow and commented: "Fascinating!"

In general, we need to raise our frequency to match the higher values of the Schumann Resonances. The wisdom traditions talk of this of being an ascension into the age of Aquarius. The higher the vibration, the closer to God or Love. So how can you bring yourself back into tune with our planetary home and raise your frequency, recalibrate your body, and continue your awakening in harmony with the times—preferably without the irksome side effects?

Sonic vitamins!

If you are ready to reset your dial, read on.

Next I will describe sonic vitamins and sound healing. Then I will describe how sound healing achieves the healing it promises.

WHAT ARE SONIC VITAMINS?

The medicine of the future will be music and sound.

EDGAR CAYCE, "FATHER OF
HOLISTIC MEDICINE"

When I first contemplated writing this book, I realized that I would be standing on the shoulders of giants—the Vedic scriptures, the Bible, the Qur'an, Pythagoras, Hans Jenny, Joseph Puleo, Leonard G. Horowitz, and Hans Cousto—to name but a few. So many luminary people go before me, some of whom I have been privileged to study with in person, via their online seminars, or through the body of work they have left in print to show inquiring minds the way. In this, I include Jonathan Goldman, Andi Goldman, Stewart Pearce, Tim Wheater, John Beaulieu, Tom Kenyon, James D'Angelo, Mark Swan, Yogi Ashokananda, Debbi Walker, and the many guests I have had the good fortune to host on my 12radio show, *Breakfast With Erica,* over many years. It is from this vast history and the extensive work of others that my concept of sound healing delivered as sonic vitamins has been developed.

When we talk of being well, we say we are in sound health. From ultrasound to corporate-funded gong bathing, tuning forks to chanting, sound healing and vibrational medicine are now coming of age. In this field, sonic vitamins are an often inexpensive and easy way to incorporate the healing benefits of sound and vibration into your daily life.

What do I mean by sonic vitamins? To understand this concept, let us consider them alongside their better-known culinary cousins, dietary vitamins. When we wish to improve our health using nutrition, we often turn to dietary vitamins to address deficiencies. The same principle applies to sonic vitamins.

Broadly speaking, all sound and vibration affects us. Just like food, what we take in can bring us health or detract from our well-being. We consume sounds from the vibrational soup in which we exist every day from our moment of birth and even before birth in the womb. While we may pay attention to what we eat, how often do we pay attention to what we take in sonically? This book is designed to guide you through some of the ways you can become aware of and utilize sound and vibration to your benefit. As dietary vitamins regulate and balance chemical and hormonal body functions, sonic vitamins can improve our health or balance deficiencies caused by stressful living. And, like dietary vitamins, sonic vitamins permeate every cell of every organ.

 Sound is a healing gift, present in every moment, freely available for all to use.

The therapeutic application of sound, music, frequency, and vibration is a natural way to treat pain and illness by stimulating the body's healing mechanisms to bring them back to balance or sound health. Sound healing (taking sonic vitamins as I like to call it), whether applied by a professional therapist or through self-administration, is simple to use and has no harmful side effects.

Before we proceed, I want to take a moment to explain the difference between sound healing and music therapy. A music therapist is usually a professional musician working with music to transcend psychological blocks. A sound therapist may also be a musician (but doesn't have to be), who applies sound and frequency for mental, emotional, physical, and spiritual enhancement. The Health Careers website for the United Kingdom explains, "Central to music therapy is the relationship that is established and developed between client and therapist. [. . .] Using music in this way, clients can create their own unique musical language in which to explore and connect with the world and express themselves. [. . .] Music therapy can be particularly helpful when emotions are too confusing to express verbally. This could be because of communication difficulty or when words are too much or not enough."[8]

Sound healing can be as individual and varied as the humans on this planet. Just as we might choose a dietary vitamin to address a particular deficiency, and then switch to another when it has done its job and we feel the need in a different area, so you may be drawn to some sonic vitamins initially, and later change your regimen to others. We all carry our own unique blueprint and vibration, so what works well for one person may not resonate so well with another. Our needs are individual and variable.

In this book, I invite you to explore your own route to sound health, choosing whichever practices strike a chord. Studying and working with healing and sound has been my passion since the 1990s. I wanted to create a place to bring together all I have learned about both and to share the wonderful possibilities for healing mind, body, and spirit that they jointly offer. Moreover, I wanted to make this vast and complex knowledge easily available for simple daily practice. Then it came to me that to ingest and absorb therapeutic sound daily is akin to taking a daily sonic vitamin.

The aim of this book is to give you tools to connect with your inner healer for guidance and to understand the power of sound that you uniquely possess in the form of your voice, affirming thoughts, and sonic intention. I will discuss various sound tools such as chakra chants, angelic vibrations, singing bowls, drums, gongs, and tuning forks. I will also include a rudimentary discussion of cymatics—the study of wave phenomena that makes sound visible.

Please also understand that sonic vitamins are your choice to create the conditions for your best holistic health, which is when your body is working efficiently, and your immune system is tuned. As with dietary vitamins, they are not a substitute for medical consultation.

You may find you wish to use all or just part of the information contained in each chapter. Whatever works for you is perfect, and you will choose exactly what your subconscious mind and divine spirit understand you need. I would also like to say here that there are no belief systems or religious doctrines attached to the therapeutic use of sound. I will, as I have just done, refer to *spirit, soul,* and *divinity* in this book. These are just semantics, words to describe the innate wisdom and highest intuition of the body that you may, or may not, connect to your wisdom tradition or spiritual practice. Whether you believe in a higher power or not, your body is sacred to you. As an angel therapist, I work with angelic vibrations and feel it would be remiss of me not to share that with you, so there is a brief section dealing with angelic vibration. However, no belief is necessary beyond a desire to work with your body's energetic intelligence howsoever you perceive it.

 Treating yourself to a daily sonic vitamin is a practice that can greatly enrich your life, bring peace where there is stress, and help you to detach from the dramas of life. Perhaps you are acquainted with some of this already, or perhaps it is new to you. Whichever is the case, I hope you will enjoy deepening your practice and nourishing your body and soul.

HOW DOES SOUND HEALING WORK?

Long before there was medicine, we healed. The body innately knows how to heal itself and we are born with that ability. Andrew Weil, M.D., an authority in integrative medicine, brainwaves, and healing, is sure that "the body knows how to heal itself."[9] We just have to give it the right instructions when it has temporarily lost its way.

In the field of quantum physics, or more specifically quantum mechanics, there is no matter. Everything is energy or vibration. In the older science of Newtonian physics, the atom was the smallest known bit of matter. Now, quantum mechanics has shown that atoms consist of even smaller particles, and at the heart of their composition is nothing—space, pure existence, and energy. The energy that each electron in an atom emits is like a wave.

As a living being, you have various layers of energy just as an atom has neutrons, protons, electrons, and quarks. In more esoteric terms, we have a physical body as well as an energetic body, the latter of which is even more susceptible to sound and vibration. We are so much more than the physical body. Our light bodies or energetic bodies surround us in layers, or energy fields. The sensation when our waves meet others is something we feel physically, mentally, and emotionally.

If we think of ourselves as being like one of those Russian Babushka dolls with many dolls nesting inside the outer later, then you have an idea of our aura.

Let us begin with the spark of divinity in the center of our physical body; that is our soul, spark of consciousness, or whatever name your wisdom tradition has called it. It is our immortality that continues when the corporal body dies. From there, we have seven layers or auric fields. Each of these auric fields has its own frequency that interacts with all the other fields and the human body. Each field is described in the following list.

1. We are acutely aware of the physical body from the moment we are born. It includes organs, bones, nerves, and sinews. We feel the pleasures and pains it creates to teach us how

to live on Earth. But perhaps we are not always so aware and tuned in to the other six nonphysical auric layers.

2. The emotional body makes up our next layer and is associated with our feelings and our moods. When it is out of tune, the whole living mechanism is thrown out of kilter. The emotional field reaches 1 to 3 inches (2.54–7.62 centimeters) from the body.

3. The mental field can reach anywhere from 3 to 8 inches (9–20 centimeters) from the body and contains our thoughts, ideas, and cognitive processes. It needs to be in balance with the emotional body to link intuition and logic.

4. Next we have the astral or causal field, which is the bridge between our physical existence and the spiritual realms. It can carry imprints of past lives.

5. The next auric field is the etheric template. It can extend 12 inches (30 centimeteters) from the body, and it is where we can connect to the spiritual realms and feelings of unconditional love and joy. It is the field where we may find clarity about life's purpose, a sense of connection to those around us, and our place in the universal scheme of things.

6. The celestial aura, or sixth field, can extend up to 2.5 feet (about 80 centimeters). This level is connected to the spiritual realm. Communication with those in the spiritual realm takes place here along with unconditional love and feelings of ecstasy.

7. And finally, the seventh layer, the ketheric or divine field, extends 3 feet (90 centimeters) and holds all the other auric fields together. It vibrates at our highest frequency and allows us to feel the oneness of creation and the universal life force that permeates all existence.

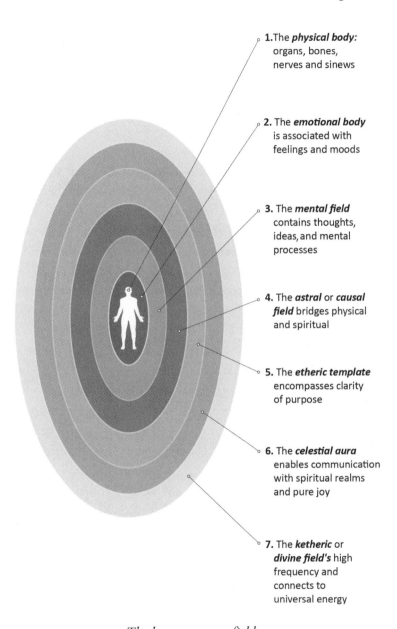

1. The *physical body:* organs, bones, nerves and sinews

2. The *emotional body* is associated with feelings and moods

3. The *mental field* contains thoughts, ideas, and mental processes

4. The *astral* or *causal field* bridges physical and spiritual

5. The *etheric template* encompasses clarity of purpose

6. The *celestial aura* enables communication with spiritual realms and pure joy

7. The *ketheric* or *divine field's* high frequency and connects to universal energy

The human energy fields
Illustration by Leonie Bunch

For optimum health, all seven fields need to be in harmony yet also play their individual role. Just as an orchestra is made up of many instruments, the beauty of a symphony is experienced when the instruments combine their multiple frequencies with the intention to create harmonic beauty, move the emotions, and thrill the heart.

You may need to retune your auric fields if you feel you have lost your sense of direction in the world or that your life lacks purpose, especially if you find negativity overwhelming you and can't seem to find balance.

 The world is a place of joy and shadows, but the one should not outweigh the other. Tuning the auric field will help you negotiate your way through life and find balance.

So how do we tune up our auric field? Each of the vitamins in this book will have a unique affect.

+ Gong bathing (Vitamin G), singing bowls (Vitamin B), or tuning forks (Vitamin F) will be particularly beneficial and have additional benefit when being directed by a trained practitioner.
+ Your own voice (Vitamins C, M, and V) is available 24/7.
+ The simple act of breathing (Vitamin B) is one of the most accessible and instant ways to reduce stress. When we breathe fully into our lower lungs, belly breathing as we did when we were babies, we increase oxygen, lower blood pressure, and bring the mind into the present moment.
+ Humming (Vitamin M, so named after the sound that is made when humming) and singing (an integral part of

many of the vitamins) have a remarkable effect both physically and on the psyche and spirit.

When we employ the power of sound, some specific effects are the stimulation of nitric oxide, the destruction of disease, and the feeling of overall harmony within the body. Each is described further below.

Nitric oxide (NO) is a molecule created when a nitrogen atom binds to an oxygen atom. NO is fundamental to all animate life on this planet, including plants. In humans, it is created in our vascular (blood) system and nerve and immune cells and is released into our tissues as a gas. It is not released in a constant stream but at regular intervals or cycles called "puffing." This regular level of NO keeps our cells balanced, relaxed, and slightly alert in order to monitor our health. When we are under attack from viruses or bacteria, our body cells increase the production of NO. This sounds the alarm and initiates a biochemical response. NO by itself can also attack to neutralize viruses, bacteria, and free radicals. Once the threat is neutralized, the body cells return to a relaxed and watchful state. NO works in six-minute puffing cycles that instruct the autonomic nervous system to hold a balance between the parasympathetic (relaxed) mode and the sympathetic (fight-or-flight) mode. When we are stressed, we remain in sympathetic mode. The result is a compromised NO puffing cycle, and in extremis, a shutdown. This can have serious consequences for our health and the cardiovascular system in particular.

Researchers use the word *spiking* to describe the stimulation or reactivation of NO puffing in cells. If stress has led to compromised NO puffing, research has shown that the application of the 128 Hz tuning fork to spike and enhance NO puffing will return the autonomic nervous system to balance and signal the natural release of antibacterial, antiviral agents on a microcellular level. Naturopathic physician John Beaulieu writes: "We experimented with the tuning forks in the lab [. . .] At first the biochemists could not believe how fast the reaction took place, or that it even took place at all. [. . .] We observed the nitric oxide spiking. [. . . .] When the nervous system comes into tune and nitric oxide is stimulated, some of the benefits attributed by researchers are: enhanced cell vitality which is the basis of anti-aging, a stabilized body metabolism that regulates digestion and body weight, an enhanced vascular flow leading to increased energy, stamina, sexual drive, enhanced memory, and a greater sense of wellbeing. Furthermore, research has demonstrated that the proper stimulation of NO acts as a preventative to the development of arteriolar sclerosis, stroke, heart attack, diabetes, Alzheimer's, depression, autoimmune disease, and cancer."[10]

Another way that sound can support health is that it can eliminate disease and other unwanted invaders of the body. Royal Raymond Rife discovered that each disease, bacterium, and virus has a unique electronic signature and vibrates at its own unique frequency and pattern. In other words, each has a sonic identity just as we all have individual fingerprints. He proposed that viruses and bacteria all have their own fields and that the field must be destroyed, or they would revive. So, he worked to create a field of resonance that would target each virus or bacterium within its specific field of sound and thus destroy it.[11]

Sound can also bring together incoherent systems into holistic resonance, harmony, and health, which impacts our psyche and spirit, benefits us physically, and helps us to tune our auric field. In physics, the word *entrainment* means that "two objects or systems that are oscillating or vibrating differently can be brought into synchronicity." It is thought that the suprachiasmatic nuclei of the brain is the master pacemaker that entrains the periphery of the body. Think of how pendulum clocks can oscillate in synchronicity when near one another. The use of specific frequencies can entrain the body, its organs, and nervous system to a state of balance, thus creating the optimum condition for healing and health.

For example, listening to music has an uplifting or calming effect on our emotional and mental state. Consider the effect of a favorite song or musical passage that evokes visions of beauty or crosses a bridge to a time when we experienced happiness in a certain place or with a person we love. Listening to or creating music can lower the heart rate and blood pressure. It can inspire us to follow our dreams or face difficult circumstances.

Sound is a bridge to other worlds. Certain sounds can transport us around the planet to oceans and forests, temples and mountain tops. The sound of rainfall can soothe and relax the mind. Drumming and rhythm have likewise been known for millennia for their effects on the human psyche and body.

As you read through this book, you will find examples of ways to employ and integrate sound in every spectrum of your daily life.

What if every word, thought, or sound you encounter in daily life is as important and powerful as the food you eat? If we are what we eat, we are also what we hear. Is your sonic diet nourishing or toxic?

How to Use This Book

FOR EASE AND SIMPLICITY OF ACCESS, I have divided this book into twelve chapters, each one centered around particular sonic vitamins. You may work through them in order or intuitively turn to one that catches your attention. Sometimes the information crosses over or is relevant to more than one vitamin. Where this occurs, I have done my best to cross-reference.

This book does not go in depth into the complexities of the vitamins, some of which have entire books dedicated to them. Where I am aware of existing references, I have listed them in the resources section at the end of this book. Here my intention is to introduce you to the many facets and possibilities of therapeutic sound with the hope that this book will act as a springboard for your own exploration.

At the start of each chapter, I have included some scientific facts and research to support the efficacy of therapeutic sound. I like to know why something works, but if you find there is too much information to take in during your first read, you can move straight to the section at the end of each chapter about how to take the sonic vitamins to begin using them.

Sonic vitamins, like their dietary counterparts, are most effective when taken daily. You may choose to focus on one area of your life where you feel a chosen vitamin is what you need, but ultimately multivitamins support a more balanced and holistic outcome. Listen to your body, and use your common sense. If you are currently on allopathic medication or under the instructions of a doctor, please do not discontinue your regimen. You may wish to discuss your choice to use vibrational medicine with your doctor and monitor your progress to see if you can become less reliant on pharmaceuticals.

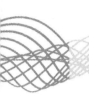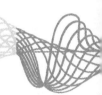

*Sonic Vitamins
for Sound Health*

VITAMIN A

Affirmations, Angels

AFFIRMATIONS

You are a community of 50 trillion cells and all of them are listening to you 24/7. What signals do you send them? The stories we tell ourselves about our worth, how we feel about ourselves, and the world and our place in it influence our auric field.

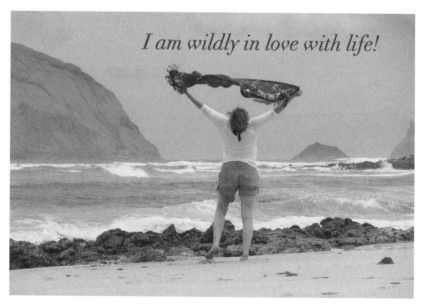

I am wildly in love with life!

Image by StuartForster.com

You lose around 300 million cells per minute: that's 50–70 billion a day. Your cells are constantly issuing instructions to renew you, so the messages you send them matter. Your miraculous body is a super generator. What a gift— living reincarnation! Tuning in to how we talk to ourselves brings us into the practice of mindfulness. Being mindful is being aware of the present moment and our actions. Like any skill, it takes practice. Just stop in this moment, right now, and ask yourself if you have been kind to yourself today. Did you wake and with your first breath thank your body for functioning beautifully through the night, your heart for beating, and your organs for clearing your system, all to get ready for the day?

Please don't wait until you feel unwell before you tune in to your body. Don't take it for granted. Take a deep breath, close your eyes to get in touch with your physical inner world, and thank your body now for being the magnificent vessel it is. Thank it for what it allows you to experience.

 Every cell in my body is doing its best to be the best it can be, right now. I am deeply grateful.

Sound healing doesn't have to be loud or vocal. Our thoughts are powerful vibrations. They resonate through our physical body and thence into our entire auric field, every sphere of which is interrelated.

Though some may prefer to use the power of thought to speak affirmations, affirmations can also be spoken aloud. Either way, it is important that you really mean what you say. The affirmation needs to come from your heart not just your head. Remember the magic of the heart's intention mentioned earlier in this book: it is 5,000 times more powerful than the brain. Now, there are people who might say, "I've tried affirmations, but they didn't work." I would ask them in reply, "How did you send them? Did you just repeat the words in your head yet secretly hold a belief that this is all mumbo jumbo? Or did you engage the power of your heart?" Also, transference works best at the lower (slower) frequency of the theta state—that's when you are just about to fall asleep, in meditation, or under hypnosis. So, I ask again, how did you send the signal? And when did you try sending it? Were you fully engaged with your heart's intention, or simply repeating words in your head while dealing with another daily task?

 Healing requires feeling.

At first, you may have to fake it if you are not used to this work and feel uncomfortable. Keep going. You will feel more comfortable in time. If you need inspiration for your affirmations or would like to work with a particular condition or injury, I refer you to Louise Hay's seminal workbook, *You Can Heal Your Life.*

Remember, your body is listening to you twenty-four hours a day. As you prepare to sleep, thank your body for everything it has done or endured that day. Ask your organs to cleanse your systems through the night so that you can start your next day as well as possible. If you have experienced difficulty in the day or are feeling unwell, send your body love as you would a child or anyone dear to you. Seriously, would you berate them for being ill? Of course not. You would nurture them, soothe them, and encourage them. Do the same for yourself!

ANGELS

You will have heard of them, of course, but not perhaps in the realm of sound healing. As I have said earlier, everything is vibration. Even if we can't see it, we most certainly feel it. If you are not sure whether angels exist or have not considered working with them to improve your well-being, I recommend you open your parameters of belief to give it a try. I do not ask you to take anything on blind faith. The aim of this book is for you to work with the vitamins and to document the experiences for yourself.

Angels are not fluffy mystical cherubs as they are often portrayed in popular art; they are mighty, cosmic energies capable of transcending dimensions, time, and space. Their power to facilitate healing is legendary. When we connect to them, our vibrational human energy fields are raised and illuminated by their vastly higher vibrational frequencies.

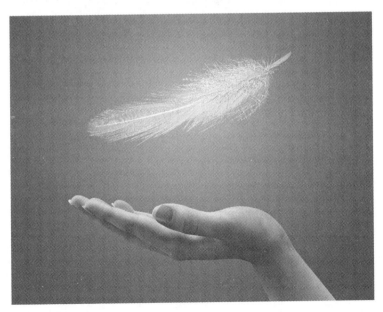

You are surrounded by angels and have been since your conception, so why haven't they stepped in to cure you? Spiritual law and being born into a world with free will means that they cannot intervene unless you summon them. The only exception is if your life is in danger and it is not your time to go. (Mine were certainly on guard during my car accident.) You don't have to tell them what to do as their overview is far wiser than ours. Simply tell them what area of your life you would like to heal.

To call them to you, you can ask them to help you by voicing your request or by asking them through the power of your thoughts. As we have already discovered, thought is vibration. You might also say or sing their names. Even if you can't see them, they will be there in an instant.

Often, they will leave "calling cards" such as little white feathers or small coins on the ground, or you will see the same message three times during your week. For example, if you are asking for advice about what to do in a situation you might see an article in the newspaper, or overhear a conversation, or hear a song on the radio. Once, I was sitting in an outside café by a fishing dock and, after asking this question, the radio on board one of the boats suddenly seemed to be have been amplified and the words: "There will be an answer, let it be" from the well-known Beatles song captivated my attention. It was, of course, the perfect advice.

⊙ Ways to Take Vitamin A

Affirmations to Heal Your Body

Affirmations can be expressed aloud or thought in one's mind. Remember, the most important aspect of "speaking" an affirmation is that your words and their power come from the heart.

- If you desire change within your body, speak internally to the part of yourself you wish to change. If you want your hair to grow luscious and long, talk to it, envision it touching your spine, and mentally feel it swish as you turn your head. Mentally say: *I love the feel of my gorgeous, long hair. It makes me so happy. Thank you, every follicle on my head, each one of you is loved and valued.*
- Pick an area of your body that you wish to heal and write an affirmation to help. For example: I love and accept all my body, just as it is, especially my . . . (whatever part of your body image you struggle with). Now place this affirmation on your mirror and say it aloud every time you pass by and every time you look into your reflection. Include your name for extra power. Your name, as you will see in Vitamin N, is unique to you and therefore holds special power that is unique to you as well. If you were to add your name, you would write and say: I, INSERT YOUR NAME, love and accept my body . . .

Affirmations to Change Your Life

Below are some additional affirmations I have found helpful. There is no limit to the number of affirmations you can use, and you can create your own to work on whatever area you have identified. Speak or think the following:

- I trust in the process of life, knowing I am supported and loved at every moment.
- Life loves me, and I am abundantly supported.
- My income is constantly increasing. I see opportunity wherever I turn.

To heal an emotional wound from a relationship or a self-inflicted lack of self-belief, try these affirmations:

- All my relationships begin and end with me. I love and accept myself unconditionally. I forgive those who have wounded me by thought, word, or deed, and in so doing, I set myself free. I was born from love. I am love. I love. I am loveable.

- I stand in awareness of this present moment. Whatever is past is gone. In this moment, I have the power to create my future. I gather together all the lessons of the past as my foundation, and I build my future on the vision of my heart.

You know yourself better than anyone on Earth. Create some of your own affirmations. Always project a positive outcome. So rather than saying "I want to change my high blood pressure," instead, say, "My body is in good health with perfectly balanced blood pressure." Focus on the outcome you desire instead of the problem. It's time to choose to love and take care of yourself.

Angelic Guidance

You have at least two guardian angels and there are a multitude more you can call on. All angels can help with everything; however, some, like the archangels, have areas of speciality, and in addition to your personal guardian angels, you can always call on the power of the mighty archangels. If you are not sure which one to choose, start with Archangel Michael, who I like to refer to as the "office manager" of archangels. Just tell him what you wish to focus on, and he will bring in the appropriate help. You can think or verbalize the affirmations spoken to the archangels. However, your voice is a powerful sound tool and will amplify your request.

- Call on Archangel Michael, who helps us with our life's purpose and gives us courage to make life decisions that release old patterns. He can also vacuum the auric field and energy centers (see Vitamin C, chakras) to clear negative associations and attachments.

Say: "Dear Archangel Michael, please help me to understand my unique purpose in life. Please clear my aura and energy centers and clearly show me the right path for me with signs, written words, and the words I hear. Thank you."

For more specific requests, you could try calling on Uriel, Chamuel, and Raphael to help heal emotional wounds, howsoever they manifest in the body.

- Uriel heals our attachment to the wound. (The true meaning of the word *resentment* is from the Latin *sentire*, "to feel." When we revisit or "re-sent" a grievance over and over, we empower it. It is like picking at a wound: doing so prevents healing.)

  Say: "Dear Archangel Uriel, please help me to release my attachment to past events that I revisit in anger, jealousy, rage, or indignation. Open my heart and release my grip on the memories of events that cause me pain, knowing that this release will set me free. Thank you."

- Chamuel works with unconditional love as a balm to our pain.

  Say: "Dear Archangel Chamuel, please step into my heart's center. Pour the power of unconditional love onto my pain, soothing away sorrow with the knowledge that only love is real, and everything else is passing illusion. Thank you."

- Raphael works to clear the heart and lungs, which often manifest illness when we are distressed. Lungs hold our grief and sadness. If you are working through loss, call on Raphael to help you acknowledge your pain and release it.

  Say: "Dear Archangel Raphael, please bathe my physical heart center and body with the energy of your green healing light to raise my vibration back into harmony and happiness. Thank you."

- To build and empower a new life path or personal initiative, call upon Archangel Metatron. The angelic ambassador of prioritization, organization, focus, and motivation, Metatron wields angelic alchemy on disorganization, helping those who call upon him to transform chaos to order while making the process practically effortless. This archangel is absolutely awesome in this regard! He is one of only two archangels to have lived a mortal life (the other is his spiritual brother, Sandalphon, who transports our prayers and affirmations to the universe). They both understand what it takes to surmount the challenges of being human.

  Say: "Dear Archangel Metatron, please help me with the power of your sacred geometry to organize and complete my project (name the exact nature of the endeavor) to create the perfect outcome at the perfect time. Thank you."

  Metatron can even come to your aid during a traffic jam or train delay. Say: "Dear Archangel Metatron, please help me to arrive at my destination on time. Thank you."

Another way to work with the angelic vibrations is by listening to or being treated by a sound healer using special tuning forks called angel tuners. These are very high frequency forks tuned on the Pythagorean scale (see Vitamin F, frequency).

~~~~~~~~~~~~~~~~~

Breath, Bowls

BREATH

Breath is the mainstay of life, and the quality of each breath makes a huge difference to our well-being. And yet, few of us pay attention to our respiration unless there is a problem. Without breath, we can make no utterance, no vocal vibration, but breath is so much more than that. As well as being our physical support, breath is also a bridge between our body, mind, and spirit. It can re-energize us, revitalize us, and simultaneously create space to connect with our mind and inner spiritual or essential self. From the standpoint of the ancient Indian Vedic philosophy, it powers our energy channels.

Focusing on breath helps us to connect to the world in which we exist. The Earth breathes. You can watch her on Youtube in a video that uses a compilation of images from NASA.[1] The oceans ebb and flow; that is their way of breathing with the Earth.

Breathing was your first act as an individual on this planet, and it will be your last. When we breathe in, we inspire; that is to say, we take in life and a new beginning with every breath. It is the root of the word *inspiration*. When we share ideas with others, we breathe together; we conspire (hence the word *conspiracy*). And finally, as the last breath of life force leaves us, we expire. Breathing is the most important thing we ever do.

Learning to breathe properly, bringing in the maximum nourishment of oxygen and releasing waste products, is one of the most powerful ways of replenishing and healing our body and mind. For this reason, breathing is the foundation for yogic practice. Indeed, there is a yogic practice dedicated solely to breath and listening to our inner sound (see Vitamin N, nada yoga). Our state of breath is a good indicator of our state of mind. For example, when we are relaxed, we breathe slowly; when we are tense or afraid, we breathe into the upper part of the chest and our breath is restricted; when we are grief-stricken or panicking, we hyperventilate. If we are aware of breath and know how to use it wisely, it can help us to make the best judgments in difficult situations and thus save us from making rash or knee-jerk decisions. A study of correct breathing technique is essential for any orator, singer, or musician, and good breath control is the essential groundwork for effective voice work and chanting (see Vitamin C).

Breathing also interacts with the body's nervous system. The body's levels of stress hormones are regulated by the autonomic nervous system (ANS), which has two components that balance each other, the sympathetic nervous system (SNS) and the parasympathetic nervous system (PNS). The SNS turns up your nervous system. It helps us handle what we perceive to be emergencies and is in charge of the fight-or-flight response. The PNS turns down the nervous system and helps us to be calm. It promotes relaxation, rest, sleep, and drowsiness by slowing our heart rate, slowing our breathing, constricting the pupils of our eyes, increasing the production of saliva in our mouth, and so forth. The PNS is influenced by a further benefit of deep breathing, the activation of the vagus nerve, which is responsible for creating a relaxation response. The vagus nerve is the longest of the cranial nerves, extending from the brainstem to the abdomen by way of multiple organs including the heart, esophagus, and lungs. The vagus nerve controls the parasympathetic nervous system (PNS), which controls your relaxation response.

The vagus nerve uses the neurotransmitter acetylcholine to communicate with the diaphragm. In addition to acetylcholine being calming and relaxing, new research has found that acetylcholine puts a major brake on inflammation in the body. In other words, stimulating your vagus nerve sends acetylcholine throughout your body, not only relaxing you but also turning down the fires of inflammation related to negative effects of stress.[2]

Exciting new research has also linked stimulation of the vagus nerve to improved neurogenesis, the development of nerves, nervous tissue, and the nervous system. Stimulation of the vagus nerve also increases brain-derived neurotrophic factor, a super fertilizer for your brain cells, repairs brain tissue, and supports actual regeneration throughout the body.[3] For example, Theise et al. have found that stem cells are directly connected to the vagus nerve. "Activating the vagus nerve can stimulate stem cells to produce new cells and repair and rebuild your own organs," they say.[4]

If you are unsure whether you are breathing fully into your belly as you did when you were a baby with no self-consciousness about how you looked, try the following exercise.

☽ How to Take a Deep Breath

Lie on your back on the floor. You can support your head with a small folded towel if you wish, but it is better if your head is in contact with the floor so that your neck and throat are not tipped forward. Note how you are feeling—perhaps tired, or edgy, or neutral.

Make a fist with both hands and place them knuckle-to-knuckle just below your breastbone. Consciously take a breath only into your upper chest. You will see that your knuckles are stationery and still together.

Now set your intention to breathe deeply into your belly. Allow your abdomen to rise as your diaphragm lowers and breath enters the lower lungs. Keep breathing as the air goes into your back and finally into the upper chest cavity. Hold for a second or so, and then breathe out as fully as you can.

Did your knuckles part a little way? If they did, you are breathing correctly.

If you find this too difficult in the beginning, place a light book on your stomach, and practice breathing so that the book rises up a little.

Take five or ten good breaths and then rest, breathing as you normally would. Check in with yourself to see how you feel physically, mentally, and emotionally.

Can you see how being able to do this, at will, whenever and wherever you desire, would bring instant benefits to any situation? As you expand your practice, listen to your breath. Does it catch in your throat? If so, mindfully open your throat or adjust your position so that the airway is straightened and not restricted. Think of your posture when you are standing or sitting. Do you restrict your lungs and airway?

Now that you are aware of your breath, try to bring that awareness into everyday life. When you are sitting at traffic lights or waiting for public transport, rather than fretting over the wait, take your focus to your breath. Is it shallow and tense? In those stationary moments, check in with yourself and realign your well-being with slow, full breaths. Do this as often as life gives you moments of pause. Supermarket queues often present an opportunity to practice this!

When at rest, the average adult breathes 12–20 times a minute, that's a potential 17,000–30,000 breaths a day! What a difference we could make to our lives and well-being if we had 30,000 B vitamins per day!

BOWLS

Singing bowls have been used from antiquity to bring harmony and healing to the human body and spirit. In the 1990s and early part of the twenty-first century, Dr. Mitchell Gaynor, director of medical oncology at the Center for Integrative Medicine at the Weill Cornell Medical Center in New York, famously used singing bowls in the treatment of his patients. He once remarked that if he had been told when he began his medical training that he would be using singing bowls as a therapy, he would have called the person who said so crazy. Nevertheless, his results are well documented.[5]

Traditional Tibetan singing bowls (also known as rin gongs, Himalayan bowls, or suzu gongs) are made from seven or sometimes eight metals (a bronze alloy containing copper, tin, zinc, iron, silver, gold, and nickel). The existence of singing bowls dates back to the time of the historical figure Buddha Shakyamuni (560–480 BCE). The tradition was brought from India to Tibet along with the teachings of the Buddha by the great tantric master Padmasambhava in the eighth century CE. Antique bowls are greatly coveted and are, as a result, expensive. However, singing bowls are still handcrafted today using traditional techniques, or they may

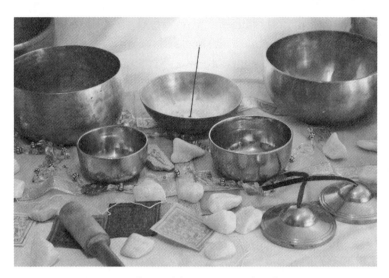

Traditional brass singing bowls

be sand cast and machine lathed. Modern bowls are far more affordable. They are often decorated with religious iconography, spiritual motifs, symbols such as the Tibetan mantra *Om Mani Padme Hum,* images of Buddhas, or the Ashtamangala (the eight auspicious Buddhist symbols).

Singing bowls vary in size and come in a variety of tunings (see Vitamin F, frequency). When a bowl is played, it is placed on a specially designed cushion or held in the palm of an outstretched hand. To commence sound healing, the bowl is gently tapped to warm up the metal. Then, with an even pressure, a specially designed mallet is rubbed clockwise around the outside edge of the rim of the bowl (like running a finger around the rim of a wine glass) to create a note. Best practice uses a full arm movement, just like stirring a big kettle of soup, and keeps the mallet straight up. Again, it's not a wrist movement as the wrist stays straight; it's an arm movement. The bowl will begin to sing its key note and all the harmonics of that scale.

(When a note is played on a musical instrument, what we are actually hearing is the fundamental pitch, which is the pitch or tone being produced by the instrument. What we think we are hearing as a single note is actually a series of frequencies that make up the rich "color" of a note. You may have heard singers, especially when using voice to chant and heal, talk about creating overtones.)

In addition to the traditional Tibetan bowls, there are crystal singing bowls. Crystal singing bowls were originally a product of the computer industry, which used quartz crucibles to grow computer chips and other components within them starting in the 1990s. More recently, quartz bowls have been enhanced with other gemstones, such as ruby and rose quartz, as well as precious metals, such as gold and silver. Crystal singing bowls are made from pure quartz silica sand. The sand is dropped into a centrifugally spinning mold, and at the proper instant, in the center of that mold, there is an electric arc torch, which is ignited to four thousand degrees centigrade. This process fuses the individual grains into one whole. This is why the interior of the bowl is smooth, and the exterior is granular and sparkly as tiny quartz grains. The bowl is then configured by sanding down the outside or trimming the bowl's height until the required note or frequency is found.

Some crystal bowls are clear. Some are frosted. Clear bowls are lighter, more expensive, and play best when held in the hand. Crystal bowls can be programmed, as crystal is able to hold, transmit, and receive thoughtforms. Quartz crystal is fundamental to the motherboards of all computers, one piece responsible for holding a computer's memory, along with completing many other tasks. "In technical terms, quartz is piezoelectric, meaning it can transform energy from one form to another," explains

John Swain, a physicist at Northwestern University. As we have already seen earlier in this book, the frequency of thoughts can be picked up and used by sensors to control objects on a computer screen. This is the mechanism that allows us to transfer our intention into any sized crystal. A large crystal bowl has the potential to become a powerful tool.[6]

Crystal bowls combine several treatment modalities: sound healing, crystal healing, and healing with light and color. These properties can be further enhanced by the power of focused intention and voice (such as those described in Vitamin A, affirmation).

Sound healing works on the principle that everything in our universe is energy that has a vibration. If you watch an activated Tibetan or crystal singing bowl with water inside it, you will see that the water agitates in waves and patterns. The human body is approximately 70 percent water, so the vibrations of the singing bowl have the same effect on us at a deep cellular level.

The frequency at which we habitually vibrate is called resonance. Different sounds resonate with different organs and parts of the body. The law of resonance states that when one energy system encounters another similar system, their vibrations must come into the state of resonance, or harmonic vibration. This process is often referred to as entrainment or synchronicity. Sound has been scientifically proven to have an effect on our autonomic, immune, and endocrine systems in addition to the neurotransmitters in our brain. When an organ in the body is out of harmony and not working as it should, its sound pattern will be distorted. It is in a state of disharmony or disease. The reintroduction of the right sound pattern will help it realign and return to harmony and health.

HOW THE BODY RELATES TO SPECIFIC FREQUENCIES
AND MUSICAL NOTES

Organ of the Body	Frequency (Hz)	Note
Blood	321.9	E
Adrenals	492.8	B
Kidney	319.88	E♭
Liver	317.83	E♭
Bladder	352	F
Intestines	281	C#
Colon	176	F
Lungs	220	A
Gall Bladder	164.3	E
Stomach	110	A
Pancreas	117.3	C#
Muscles	324	E
Bone	418.3	A#
Brain	315.8	E♭
Fat Cells	295.8	C#

In addition to targeting specific body parts, when a practitioner or individual plays a singing bowl, the sound calms and centers mind and body. The vibrating bowl emits tones that set up a "frequency following response" (entrainment) which promotes a balance between the left and right brain hemispheres, which in turn bring the whole nervous system and bodily systems into balance and homeostasis.

☾ Ways to Take Vitamin B
Developing an Awareness of Breath

To stimulate body and brain function and increase vitality and the body's regenerative powers, full, deep breathing is essential. By now, if you have followed the suggested exercise earlier in this chapter, you will be aware of the feeling when you breathe fully and deeply into your abdomen, allowing the diaphragm to relax and expand downward. If you are not breathing fully, you are not experiencing life to the fullest. With regular practice, you will increase your lung capacity and your ability to inhale Vitamin B.

- Sit comfortably on a chair with your feet flat on the floor, or sit on the floor cross-legged (in lotus if you are accustomed to this pose and can maintain it comfortably). Keep your spine erect, and close your eyes and your mouth (you will be breathing through your nose) and begin by breathing normally. As you do, become aware of the three centers of breath.
    - First, take your attention to your navel, or belly button.
    - Then focus on your mid chest and rib cage.
    - And finally, shift your awareness to your upper chest.
- As you inhale, separate the intake of breath into three components: breathe into your navel to the count of three, breathe into your midsection to the count of three (feel your ribs expand in your back), and finally, fill the top of your lungs with breath right up to the collarbone for the final count of three.
- As soon as you reach full capacity, exhale in reverse order. Empty the top of your chest first while counting to three, then your midsection, and finally, your belly. Make sure you exhale fully to completely empty the lungs.
- Repeat this pattern for ten minutes, then rest and pay attention to how you feel mentally, emotionally, and physically.

Technique to Control the Breath

You might also like to try alternate nostril breathing, *nadi shodhana*. *Nadi* means "channel" and *sodhana* means "purification," so *nadi shodhana* means "clearing the channels of circulation."

- Find a place and way to sit so that your spine is straight (either cross-legged on the floor or in a chair with your feet on the floor), and take a moment to place your focus in your heart area.

- Relax your left palm comfortably into your lap, and bring your right hand just in front of your face.

- Bring your right index finger and right middle finger to rest between your eyebrows, lightly using them as an anchor. The fingers we'll be actively using are the thumb and ring finger.

- Close your eyes, and take a deep breath through your nose. Exhale normally through your nose.

- After exhaling, close your right nostril with your right thumb. Keeping your right nostril covered, inhale through the left nostril slowly and steadily.

- Close the left nostril with your ring finger so both nostrils are held closed; retain your breath at the top of the inhale for a brief pause.

- Open your right nostril, and release the breath slowly through the right side; pause briefly at the bottom of the exhale.

- Slowly inhale through the right nostril.

- Hold both nostrils closed (with ring finger and thumb).

- Open your left nostril, and release breath slowly through the left side. Pause briefly at the bottom.

- Repeat five to ten cycles, allowing your mind to follow your inhales and exhales. These steps represent one complete cycle of alternate nostril breathing. If you're moving through the sequence slowly, one cycle should take you about 30 seconds. Breathe through five to ten cycles when you're feeling stressed, anxious, or in need of a reset button.

- Consistency is helpful, so try to match the length of your inhales, pauses, and exhales. For example, you can start to inhale for a count of five, hold for five, exhale for five, hold for five. You can slowly increase your count as you refine your practice.

Yogic tradition teaches many exercises incorporating breath. Once you are proficient with the exercises above, you might like to extend your practice by purchasing a book that deals specifically with breathing techniques that go beyond the space and scope of this book. Two books I recommend are *The Power of Relaxation* by Yogi Ashokananda and *The Power of Breath* by Swami Saradananda.

Beginning Work with Singing Bowls

If you are interested in experiencing the benefits of singing bowls, a visit to a sound healer may incorporate this type of healing, and that experience is described at the end of this chapter. There are also two possible approaches to using the power of singing bowls for self-medication at home.

+ First, there are many recordings and videos of bowls being played. To gain the most from this approach, use headphones that will direct the sound to harmonize both right and left brain hemispheres and eliminate outside interference. Although it is preferable to receive healing sound directly from the instrument, sometimes that is not possible, and listening to a recording is the next best approach.

  It has been scientifically proven that musical recordings can be vibrationally imprinted. As was described in the first chapter in the section about affirmations, thoughts are also sound waves. So, sound + intention = holistic resonance (healing). If the intention of the performer is sincere and their intention is to send healing vibration to the recording, you will take in that vibration. Use your judgement when selecting recordings and videos. If one does not resonate with you, search for another. Instinctively, you will know which one is right. You can also search for a recording of a sound bowl with a specific frequency if you wish to work with one particular body system or organ (see the chart on page 39).

- Second, you might be inspired to buy a bowl of your own. Using your own bowl ensures that you will experience the resonance firsthand; not only will you hear the notes, you will also absorb them with your body. The best way to choose a singing bowl for personal use is to fall in love with the sound. If a bowl calls to you, you'll know that's the one for you.

  Your choice may be determined by the usage. Are you looking for a bowl for meditation, grounding, or physical healing? Do you want to integrate a few bowls into an existent modality? Does using them with other instruments in a musical vein interest you? Do you wish to use them in yoga classes to bring about relaxation at the end? Are you a nurse who wants to use them with patients during your rounds? Is this a way for you to call meetings to order in the corporate setting? The answers to these questions will impact your choices. It's a good idea to know how you want to use a singing bowl before you purchase one. On that note, collecting bowls is also an organic process—one may not be enough!

Experience Professional Sound Healing

Professional sound healing entails a visit to a certified sound healer who may use a variety of sound healing instruments, including singing bowls. The bowls may be placed around you and sounded to create a sonic bath, or they may be laid directly on your body, or both. You could lie supine with a bowl on your chest and one in each upturned palm, or you may lie prone with bowls on the chakra energy points along your spine. A discussion with the sound healer will help determine your goals and needs, and the experience you receive will reflect these. Visiting a certified sound healer confers the additional benefits of many frequencies as he or she will own more bowls than the average layman. Additionally, a sound healer can imbue the bowls with healing intention as they are played, leaving you free to relax, surrender, and absorb the healing without having to focus on the practical details. To find a therapist in your area in the United Kingdom, visit the College of Sound Healing's website. In the United States, visit the Sound Healers Association website.

Cymatics, Chakras, Chanting

IN THIS CHAPTER, YOU WILL ENCOUNTER three sound healing components, which go to the heart of well-being. You become the instrument and the player.

CYMATICS

Cymatics is the science of visible sound. When a membrane becomes excited by sound, fine particles, such as salt, vibrate on a flat plate to create beautiful patterns. Many forms resemble the outlines of primal creatures from the ocean.

While cymatics is not actually a healing modality, I have decided to include additional information about cymatics in this chapter because it is so interconnected to understanding the mystical as well as the scientific underpinnings of many of the modalities.

Experiments to show the physical representation of sound began with Galileo Galilei around 1630. Robert Hooke followed suit in 1680. By the eighteenth century, German musician and physicist Ernst Chladni had consistently produced visual patterns by vibrating the surface of a membrane or plate that had been sprinkled with a fine dust. The term *cymatics* (from the Greek word *kyma* for "wave") was coined in 1967 by Hans Jenny, a Swiss physician and natural scientist who repeated Chladni's experiments by putting sand, dust, and fluids on a metal plate connected to an oscillator that could produce a range of frequencies. The particles or fluids reacted to the frequencies by organizing into geometric patterns. Jenny published the book: *Cymatics: The Study of Wave Phenomena.* Wikipedia explains that, "According to Jenny, these structures, reminiscent of the mandala and other forms recurring in nature, would be a manifestation of an invisible force field of the vibrational energy that generated it. He was particularly impressed by an observation that imposing a vocalization in ancient Sanskrit of *Om* (regarded by Hindus and Buddhists as the sound of creation) the lycopodium powder formed a circle with a center point, one of the ways in which *Om* had been represented."[1] (See also Vitamin O, *Om.*)

When the human voice intones *Om,* the image produced through vibration on a membrane covered in sand and excited by the human voice replicates the Sri Yantra, an ancient, 12,000-year-old Hindu symbol.

The Sri Yantra is said to be the original, the mother of all yantras (mystical diagrams). It is mathematically precise, based on the golden mean or phi ratio found underlying all things in nature, and featured in many great works of art, including Leonardo Da Vinci's *Vitruvian Man* and *Mona Lisa.*

From this, we can see the power of using sound and the human voice (Vitamin V), and extrapolate that the voice can be used to retune and benefit the human body and auric fields (see Vitamin A). Therein also lies the power of chanting, which we will explore later in this chapter.

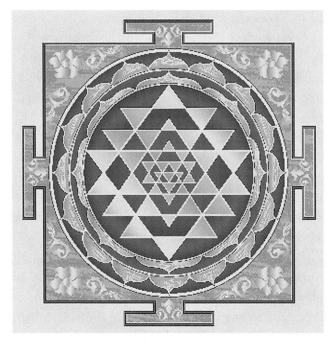

Image of the Sri Yantra mandala

CHAKRAS

In addition to the auric energy fields emanating from and surrounding the body, we have channels of energy vortices that spin at various points in the body, mostly aligning with the spine. These are called *chakras,* from the Sanskrit word *cakra* for "wheel." According to ancient Sanskrit teaching, we have 114 chakras in the body and 72,000 *nadis,* or energy channels. However, prominence is usually given to the major seven chakras.

Many modern thinkers, seers, and channelers believe that as the human race is evolving and ascending to a higher vibrational way of living that is more heart-led and compassionate, we are returning to the twelve chakra system that is said to have existed in Atlantean times. It is my personal experience that this may be true. When working with notes aligning with the seven chakras, because any note sounded is not a single frequency but a composite, we are automatically creating tones above, below, and in between, thus stimulating the wider range of chakras.

In this book, I will explore the traditional seven chakras. Each chakra has a Sanskrit name and is associated with an element, color, and musical note. However, for the purposes of sound healing, we are concerned only with the associated notes and frequencies. Note that the tones are based on the 432 Hz grid (see Vitamin F).

The tones listed can be produced using chakra tuning forks (see Vitamin F), which give the precise frequency, or you can play the notes on a musical instrument. Please be aware, however, that most pianos are tuned to 440 Hz, which is a slightly "tighter" tuning. If you use a piano to help you pitch your note with your voice or instrument, healing will still occur. If you have a digital keyboard, you should be able to adjust the tuning so that A is tuned to the frequency 432 Hz, which would be preferable.

As the chakras are part of the energetic system of the body, they first impact those corporal systems that govern the body's processes, namely the endocrine system and nervous system. If the glands of the endocrine system instruct the body in how to build and maintain itself and the nervous system governs bodily responses, it follows that balancing these systems to optimal working status will enhance the health of the body at a deep cellular level.

According to medical science, the human body completely renews itself approximately every 7 years. The cornea replaces itself every 24 hours, the skin every 14–28 days, the blood cells

CHAKRA TONES BASED ON THE 432 HZ GRID

1st Chakra **ROOT**		Grounded *NOTE C*	**128 HZ** **256 HZ** **512 HZ**
2nd Chakra **SACRAL**		Open *NOTE D*	**144 HZ** **288 HZ** **576 HZ**
3rd Chakra **SOLAR PLEXUS**		Confident *NOTE E*	**162 HZ** **324 HZ** **648 HZ**
4th Chakra **HEART**		Compassionate *NOTE F#*	**182.25 HZ** **364.5 HZ** **729 HZ**
5th Chakra **THROAT**		Expressive *NOTE G*	**192 HZ** **384 HZ** **768 HZ**
6th Chakra **THIRD EYE**		Intuitive *NOTE A*	**216 HZ** **432 HZ** **864 HZ**
7th Chakra **CROWN**		Connected *NOTE B*	**243 HZ** **486 HZ** **972 HZ**

The seven chakras with their associated notes and frequencies.
The chart shows the chakra notes based on the root note being C.
There are other chakra scales that use G as the root note.
Neither is wrong. The G root note is a more modern innovation.
A root note is the first note of a scale.

Image by Leonie Bunch

every 90 days, the bones every 6 weeks, the soft tissue every 6 months, and the dense tissue every 2–7 years. Regular fine-tuning of the chakras gives the body's network the best conditions for healthy self-renewal.

CHANTING

When I first started working with sound, I was confused about the difference between toning and chanting. I wondered if they were the same thing. I am indebted to James D'Angelo, author of *The Healing Power of the Human Voice,* whose weekend course on sound healing at Goldsmith University was my introduction to this magical work. Over the weekend, he shared the definitions that made sense of the difference for me. He said:

> Toning is the repetition of single sounds or syllables. The vowels are the essence of the sound and are stretched out longer than they would be in normal speech. They can be preceded *and/or* succeeded by consonants as in the case of toning the chakras.
>
> Chanting is actually a form of singing, characterized by the repetition of short phrases of tones, fairly narrow in range, often wedded to some kind of sacred text and done as part of a ritual.

Using your voice to talk, sing, or chant is uplifting and self-empowering. It is a joy for me to see the rise in popularity of community choirs; many have brought communities together and engaged disadvantaged and disaffected young people and adults.

By using your breath and your voice together in a chant, you raise the level of your own vibration.

Chanting, a form of vocal meditation, is practiced by many people around the world who seek greater health, a sense of well-being, enlightenment, and a connection to the divine. Chanting unites the mind, body, emotions, and breath through vocal expression. This unification can open and nurture your creativity, lower stress levels, and teach you to become fully alert and in the moment.

Some people are naturally drawn to chant while others feel awkward using their voices in such a way. We have been conditioned to think of using our voices as a performance.

When we play, chant, or sing intending to use sound for healing purposes, sound is used for entrainment not entertainment.

If you feel nervous, try chanting along with recorded chants before chanting on your own. However, know that the chanting that will resonate most deeply and beneficially for you is the chanting you do for yourself, either alone or as part of a group.

Chanting is usually performed in an ancient language, such as Tibetan, Sanskrit, Latin, or a variety of indigenous tribal languages. The reason that this tradition is so effective and, therefore, is still the basis for this mode of healing, is the effect of the shape of the mouth and the action of the tongue required in order to formulate and speak those words. There are eighty-four meridian points on the hard palate on the roof of the mouth. Each point can be stimulated by speaking or singing sacred words, and vowels in particular (see Vitamin V).

These act as a form of oral reflexology. The eighty-four meridians connect and communicate with the hypothalamus in the brain. The chanting of sacred phrases, which repeatedly impacts these sensitive points, translates into instructions to the hypothalamus to produce chemicals (neurotransmitters) that influence sleep, hunger, thirst, and body temperature. The hypothalamus is above the thalamus, which is linked to the pituitary gland, which I like to call "the leader of the endocrine orchestra." It conducts and instructs all the glands and their processes. Consciously chanting can balance our chakras and bring us into holistic resonance, or sound health.

 Using sacred syllables and chanting transcends feelings of sorrow, anger, joy, and happiness. They are all vibrational frequencies of the mind. When we chant, we lay the foundation to find balance and peace.

☺ Ways to Take Vitamin C

Become the Instrument

Now that you are aware of cymatics and the way vibration acts upon any membrane it encounters, it is easy to see why and how you are affected by targeted sound. When you use a sound healing tool, such as a singing bowl or tuning fork, or when you tone or chant, you can become the membrane that is excited by sound.

- To experience this, strike the singing bowl or turning fork.
- Guide it from the base chakra at the bottom of your spine to the crown chakra at the top of your head. Wait until the note's vibration has completely died away before you move to the next position.
- If this is physically difficult to achieve while standing, lie down, place the singing bowl or tuning fork on top of you, and strike it.

The most vital work happens as the instrument's or fork's note diminishes and releases into the body. Rest for a minute or so afterward, and review your mind and body sensations. Become your own scientist, and explore what you experienced as the cymatic membrane. What did you feel, see, or hear?

Choosing a Note to Balance the Chakras

If you look at the chart on page 49 and can identify an area of the body where you feel vulnerable or weaker, choose that note to work with. For example, if you are facing a meeting or conversation where you feel a lack of confidence about speaking, you might pick the note E for the solar plexus, which strengthens our confidence and personal power, and G for the throat chakra, which empowers us to openly express our ideas and beliefs. If you have an instrument that will help you find that note, strike it. If not, you will be able to find a note on the internet.

The note, or tone, you choose will depend your vocal range. Even if you decide to pick a vowel to chant on a random tone that seems comfortable to you, your intent will be to work on that chakra. There is more detailed instruction on how to chant sacred vowels to balance the chakras in Vitamin V.

You may also wish to purchase your own set of chakra tuning forks that will be fine-tuned to reproduce the exact frequencies of each chakra.

Chanting Basics

Good news! You don't have to sit in lotus position like a monk to chant!

- Either sitting or standing, assume a stable upright position with shoulders dropped. To begin, your arms can be relaxed at your sides or in prayer position at the heart. If sitting, place the palms facing upward in a cupped position in your lap. Make sure that you can get your feet flat on the floor. If lying down, support your head and neck with something soft. Allow your shoulders to relax and soften into the floor and your arms to relax at your side at the start.

- Place the hands lightly on the body to direct sound to the appropriate chakra. For the throat, cup your hands just below your jaw. For your third eye, put your palms gently over your eyes. For the crown chakra, place the hands just above either ear with your fingers over the top of your head.

- Tone slowly and rhythmically. You do not have to tone all seven chakras in each session. You may choose to concentrate on one area where you feel you most need the healing (refer to the chart on page 49 or see below for more ideas).

- Ten minutes is my recommended maximum amount of time to spend on any one chakra if you've chosen to work with a single chakra. If toning through all the chakras, aim for a maximum of thirty minutes.

Most chants are vocal, but it is also possible, and sometimes useful, to chant internally, or without creating sound. I have found motionless, silent chanting particularly effective when sitting in a public place where it would be inappropriate to be vocal but where you may wish to diffuse fear or tension, for example, in a dentist's waiting room!

Extending Your Chanting Practice

Once you are comfortable with toning notes, why not extend your practice to chant a phrase? There are many available. Some are simple, and some more challenging to learn.

If you are new to chanting, begin with something simple. The ultimate simple chant is, of course, *Om*. This chant is so powerful it has a chapter in this book all to itself, Vitamin O.

Chanting vowels is also powerful. You will find information on vowels and their meaning in Vitamin V.

For a first phrase to chant, let's start with *Sat Nam* (pronounced "sat" like I sat down, and "nam" rhyming with jam), which means "truth is my identity." Silently repeating *Sat Nam* is the route to connect to our inner world; it turns on our inner light and helps us to trust and listen to our intuition. Being able to trust ourselves and allow our inner truth to guide us in our daily choices is the road to self-mastery and peace.

- Start out by mentally preparing. Inhale and focus on the syllable *Sat*, then exhale and focus on *Nam*.
- Once you feel you have your focus, you can start to chant the two words vocally on the exhale. Inhale while focusing on the truth in your heart, exhale vocalizing *Sat Nam*.

When you are comfortable with mentally chanting *Sat Nam*, try both mentally and vocally chanting *So Ham* (pronounced "so-hum"), meaning "I am that." *That* in this case means "all creation, the creator, and the oneness with all life in the universe." In the ancient Hebrew text the Torah, when Moses asked God for a name, the creator replied *ehyeh asher ehyeh:* "I am that I am."

So Ham allows us to focus the "thinking mind" on the mystery of being and the interdependence with all life on this Earth and throughout the cosmos. It unifies the feminine and masculine in creation. The two seed syllables represent the yin and the yang. *So* is yin (feminine) and *Ham* is yang (masculine).

- As before, begin by chanting internally. Inhale to *So,* and exhale to *Ham*. In addition to working with the perspective of yin and yang, as you progress with this chant you can consider other aspects. This creates a third healing projection to consider. *So* on the inhale brings in air, cold air; *Ham* on the exhale expels warm air. Focusing on *So* during the inhale is mental; focusing on *Ham* during the exhale is emotional. You inhale spirit with *So*; you release matter while you exhale and think of *Ham*.

- Maintain your attention to your breath on the inhale, and feel how it expands you as you receive the breath of life.

- On the exhale, experience giving back. Perhaps imagine the trees who thrive on carbon dioxide as you breathe out. As you practice chanting, you are also working with Vitamin B, breath.

- When you have done this for five minutes, add a vocal dimension, toning *So Ham* on the exhale to give back to creation. Inhale and accept healing. Recall that when toning, one should really stretch the vowels.

If you would like a slightly longer vocal phrase, try chanting the Sanskrit mantra *Om Mani Padme Hum* (pronounced "ohm-mah-nee-pahd-may-hum" ["hum" is "oo" as in the word *book*]). This mantra has many depths of translation. The most common is "The jewel of the lotus resides in my heart." It is said that all of the teachings of Buddha are contained in the mantra. That concept is hard to fathom, but it is helpful to have some idea of the intention when chanting this mantra. As we have seen earlier, intention is important when using sound healing. Tomes have been written on the meaning of this mantra; however, a very simplified interpretation is: *Om* invokes the creator. *Mani*, the jewel, is the divine that dwells in the heart that is *Padme*, the lotus. *Hum* represents our individual self, a spark of divine consciousness. Another helpful perspective I was given by a Tibetan master is that this sacred mantra is the embodiment of the qualities of understanding and loving kindness, transformational and purifying virtues that address our imbalances of nature as human beings.

- To prepare, in your mind find a comfortable slow rhythm. I sometimes feel my pulse on my wrist and synchronize with that. It is a useful exercise to intentionally slow down as you practice and then check to see if your pulse responds similarly.
- Pick a single note and intone it. Don't be shy. This is not about performance; this is about bringing the mind and body together. Hold the opening *Om* for two beats, give the rest one beat, and finish with two beats for the final *Hum*. As you gain confidence there are many versions of this chant on the internet to experiment with.
- Some people recite or chant this mantra many thousands of times a day as part of their daily practice. However, chanting this mantra for even five minutes will have great benefits on your peace of mind and your ability to be compassionate with yourself and others.

Combining Chanting and Drumming

And finally, if you wish to incorporate some Vitamin C with Vitamin D (drumming) try this Arapaho Native American chant depicting wolves' mating calls. Chant *Woa Yea* in sections of three as shown on the next page. This would be a good chant to try in a chanting circle, possibly with a drum rhythm and rattles.

Someone in the circle should be designated to signal, with fingers held up, the final repetition of one set (18 words) to bring the practice to a close. Vary the rhythm, feel it, and have fun! Again, think of it in sections of three:

Woa Woa Woa
Woa Woa Woa
Woa Woa Woa
Yea Yea Yea
Yea Yea Yea
Yea Yea Yea

For more information on drumming, turn to the next chapter, Vitamin D.

VITAMIN D

Drumming, Didgeridoo

NOW THE JOURNEY INTO SOUND gets percussive and primal. Even making the vocal sound of the letter *D—duh, duh, duh*—pulses the diaphragm. The drum and the didgeridoo belong together as their sound affects the body like a vibrational sonic massage. Who doesn't like a massage?

DRUMMING

Drumming is phenomenal. Stimulating! Empowering! It's a life force! Drumming is a natural compulsion. Whether it is done with the fingers when nervous or when tapping along with a beat on the radio, drumming is a natural human impulse and one that is growing in popularity. Plato said, "Rhythm and harmony enter most powerfully into the inner most part of the soul and lay forcible hands upon it, bearing grace with them, so making graceful him who is rightly trained." As another anonymous drummer once said, "I play drums. What's your superpower?"

In nearly all cultures, both past and present, the drum is used as an instrument of healing, and nearly every culture on Earth has some form of drumming tradition. From the ancient traditions of the Celts and Druids to the Minianka healers of West Africa, the shamans of Siberia, the Aborigines of Australia, and the Native American tribes, rhythm has been used for thousands of years to address a number of health issues. Many shamans use the drum to take their initiates on a journey into the Earth and altered states of consciousness. Drumming is beneficial both to receive and to perform. It is a universal language that transcends gender, race, age, and nationality.

Researchers have found that if a drum beat frequency of three to four beats per second is sustained for at least fifteen minutes, it will induce significant trance states in most people, releasing our hold on the external world and opening the pathway to receive healing.[1] This is referred to in Zen Buddhist and Native American teaching as becoming a hollow bone, a conduit for spirit and healing. In this shamanic teaching, the drum aids us in clearing away anything that could possibly clog the bone of our spirit and mind. Meditative practice is an important part of the ongoing task of keeping our insides clean. This form of meditation also facilitates a transcendent state of unity consciousness with all that is. All we have to do is follow the beat. Drumming is a nonverbal way of expressing ourselves through sound and vibration. And it gets us moving. The word *rhythm* in Greek, *rhythmos,* means "to flow." Used therapeutically, drumming is a path of healing that guides us into experiencing the flow of our mind and emotions, so we may grow to experience more of our soul.

Because rhythmic drumming is also meditative, it induces relaxed mental states that reduce anxiety and tension. Drumming combined with deep breathing and visualization techniques offers even more stress reduction benefits. The DNA switches that are turned on with stress can be reversed with creative musical expression. In other words, by doing something as simple as drumming, biological benefits occur at the cellular level. Stress is a legacy from when stress hormones prompted us to fight or flee danger. In today's society, we experience anger, frustration, or fear, but instead of reacting, we are often forced by social conditioning to contain and internalize these feelings. While this may prevent a socially unacceptable outburst, the hormones are not switched off and remain circulating in our veins where they cause accelerated heart rate, higher blood pressure, and mental anxiety. Ideally, we need strong physical activity to disperse them. If you need to vent, what better way than to hit something, like a drum?

Drum therapy has successfully been used with patients and others suffering from emotional traumas including post-traumatic stress disorder. Drumming can help people express and address emotional issues. The mechanism behind this is that the physical stimulation of striking something removes blockages and produces emotional release. Furthermore, sound vibrations resonate through every cell in the body, stimulating the release of negative cellular memories. In addition, research suggests that drumming serves as a distraction from pain and grief. Specifically, drumming promotes the production of endorphins, the body's own morphine-like painkillers, and can thereby help to control emotional pain.[2]

Drum circles also provide an opportunity for participants to feel connected with others, gain a sense of interpersonal support, and connect with their spirit at a deeper level. Group drumming alleviates self-centeredness, isolation, and alienation. There are great benefits to feeling connected to others, especially those in similar situations.

The current popularity of drumming and participation in drum circles seems to be driven by a human need to reconnect with the beat and vibrations of life. Drumming is also one of those rare physical activities that can have both profound and subtle effects on the entire person. Research demonstrates the benefits of recreational music-making with the drum, including:

+ improved aerobic and cardiovascular system
+ strengthened immune system
+ improved mood and reduced burnout of workers under stress
+ reversed ravages of stress at the cellular level
+ reduced anxiety, depression, and feelings of loneliness

A recent medical research study indicates that drumming boosts the immune system. According to neurologist Barry B. Bittman, M.D., medical director for the Mind Body Wellness Center, the study demonstrates that group drumming actually increases cancer-killing white blood cells, which help the body fight cancer and other viruses.[3]

In addition to boosting the immune system, drumming might also help you lose weight! Bittman says, "Our preliminary testing of aerobic protocols, for example, found that by just using hand drums and moving to the beat, people burned a substantial number of calories—averaging 270.4 calories in a half-hour—with a much lower perceived exertion." In other words, people were having so much fun playing on a drum that they did not feel that they were exercising. By engaging both mind and body in the production of music, holistic healing was enabled. "People who cannot move to the music can play at their own pace; those who are not ambulatory can just drum," Bittman explains. "All the participants in the preliminary research were laughing and smiling and no one stopped to rest. This is the key—connect people to music physically and mentally, and the results are positive."[4]

If we extend the concept of fitness beyond a physical workout it is clear that we must also focus on mental, emotional, and spiritual health, also known as wellness.

The connection between the human pulse and that of nature—manifested by rhythmically beating a drum with the hands—is a recurring theme not only among indigenous peoples but also among others who find themselves drawn to drumming and drum circles. International bestselling author Dr. Christiane Northrup explains, "drumming is a great workout for your brain and actually can make you smarter because when you drum you access your entire brain. Research shows that the physical transmission of rhythmic energy to the brain actually synchronizes the left and right hemispheres. So, when the logical left hemisphere and the intuitive right hemisphere of your brain begin to pulsate together, your inner guidance system—or intuition—becomes stronger."[5]

And listening to drum sounds regularly can have the same effect as drumming itself. Like the Indian proverb says, "A good drummer listens as much as he plays." The sound of drumming generates new neuronal connections in all parts of the brain. The more connections that can be made within the brain, the more integrated our experiences become. This leads to a deeper sense of self-awareness.

Drumming also appears to synchronize the lower areas of the brain (responsible for nonverbal functions) with the frontal cortex (responsible for language and reasoning). This integration produces feelings of insight, clarity, and certainty. For these reasons, therapeutic drumming may be a powerful tool in helping retrain the brain. It has been shown to benefit people with ADHD as well as those who have some level of damage or impairment; for example, people who have had a stroke or who have Parkinson's. Furthermore, group drumming and drum therapy is currently being used to treat people with brain injuries, physical injuries, arthritis, addictions, and more.

Finally, drumming can induce a natural "high" by increasing alpha brain waves. When the brain changes from beta waves (concentration) to alpha waves, you feel calm and relaxed. Alpha waves can also produce feelings of well-being and even euphoria, which may help people who suffer from mental illness, such as depression and anxiety. This same alpha activity is associated with meditation and other integrative modes of consciousness.

So, it seems that medical experts and sound therapists are in synch; we all agree that drumming is fun, and it's good for you!

DIDGERIDOO

Alongside the drum, the didgeridoo is one of the oldest instruments in the world. Most associated with the Aboriginal tribes of the Northern Territory of Australia, a traditional didgeridoo was a fallen eucalyptus branch that had been hollowed out by termites. The nooks and crannies created inside the didgeridoo during this process give the sound produced its extraordinary and otherworldly amplification as it travels from the player's lips to the instrument's exit. Similar sonic tubes were known by the Central American Mayan tribes whose instruments were made from fallen yucca or agave. Didgeridoos are both pitched and percussive; that is to say, they have a fundamental note depending on the size of the bore and can be pulsed to sound like a drum. Therefore, they can be made to keep a bass rhythm or sing and speak. A skilled player can evoke kangaroos hopping along in the bush, the howl of dingoes in the night, and the calling of birds across the outback. The didgeridoo is designed to connect us to our natural roots and transport us to other realms.

Traditionally, in addition to being used with sonic intent to draw participants together and into a meditative trance state in tribal ritual, they were played nearby someone who was sick. The benefits of didgeridoo are twofold in that they benefit the player as well as the listener.

First, playing a didgeridoo requires constant deep breathing (Vitamin B), which expands the lung capacity, strengthens the diaphragm, and instills a strong sense of rhythm. In studies by the University of Queensland, it has been found to be very beneficial to people with asthma as playing mimics the Buteyko breathing technique used to control asthma.[6] Furthermore, a Swiss study has demonstrated an improvement in people who have sleep apnea, a condition in which breathing stops and starts during sleep, sometimes with serious consequences. This study found that playing the didgeridoo strengthens the pharyngeal muscles, (the muscles of the throat) as well as the muscles of the tongue that are implicated in loud snoring and sleep apnea.[7]

Second, listening to the sound and vibrations of a didgeridoo has a calming effect on the nervous system and also affects the physical body. The ancient vibrations that come through even the most modern didgeridoo help listeners enter a deep state of relaxation or trance. The didgeridoo produces a low-pulsed frequency that we hear and feel. It has the potential to heal tissue, particularly bone, while also unlocking energetic blocks. Current research shows improvement to bone, muscle, and hormonal balance. The didgeridoo creates infrasound and ultrasound, frequencies outside our normal range of hearing. Even though we can't hear them, our bodies are nourished by them. The didgeridoo could be said to be the sonic equivalent of acupuncture or a qi gong power wash. Like these healing methods, it frees up blocked energy meridians. At low frequency, the sound of the didgeridoo is concussive; it is a sound wave that you feel rather than hear. Anyone who has heard a live didgeridoo will tell you that the impact is otherworldly, taking them beyond their daily experience of life.

♪ Ways to Take Vitamin D

Drum Your Emotions

If you are feeling upset or agitated but not sure why and find yourself taking your mood out on others, use the most basic form of drumming available to you. Become truly primal. Hit something! This advice comes with a caveat: hit something in a way that is therapeutic and safe. The best thing I have found is a pillow.

- Go somewhere, preferably alone where you will not be watched and can really "let rip." Begin to punch the pillow slowly and with force.
- What is behind your feelings may come to you immediately. If not, keep going. Make some noise, shout, growl, or cuss.
- After a while, you might still feel annoyed, but any real anger will have dissipated along with your stress hormones. Humans usually only stay truly angry for fifteen minutes. Once you have "let it go" you can start to think calmly about your experience and how you would like to respond.

Clap It Out

One form of drumming we overlook, yet is percussive and so belongs here, is the sound we make when we "drum" our hands together—clapping. The sound of clapping is associated with approbation and elation. Being among an audience applauding is uplifting. If you have ever had the good fortune to receive applause you know how empowering it feels. Clapping is a glorious opportunity to show appreciation and gratitude that extends beyond theatrical performance. This was amply demonstrated when we stood together during the COVID-19 pandemic to show sonic appreciation for the dedication and courage of medical staff and essential workers. Not only did it lift their spirits, the collective effort brought together households, streets, and communities where daily pressures of life had led to distance and indifference. Always take the opportunity to applaud, particularly remembering to clap for yourself when you feel you deserve it.

Clapping your hands together is also a wonderful way to transform the energy of a room.

- Clap in each corner to disburse stagnant energy.
- Clap to clear the air if there has been discord.
- Fling open a window and clap around the room to chase the energy out of the space in order to make room to usher in fresh air and energy.

It is such a simple practice and yet a form of sound healing that can make a difference to a room or home. Try it and feel the change!

Additional Ways to Experience the Power of the Drum

- Listen to drumming. There are some excellent recordings of therapeutic drums available. Allow yourself to move, to flow with the rhythm, and to be as expressive as you like. You may feel like joining in by drumming on a table or yourself.
- Enjoy a sonic massage from a sound healing practitioner who uses drums.

- Join a drumming circle. Circles in any kind of gathering are always a powerful way to amplify the desired benefits of the group. In drumming, the energy flows around the room and forms a sonic pyramid in the center. The action of drumming, as discussed earlier, is meditative and healing. Simultaneously, you receive the vibration in every cell of your body and may find participation in a drum circle to be destressing, soothing, and uplifting.
- Go out into nature, which is healing in and of itself, and drum a rhythm on a log or rock.

Drift Away with the Sound of the Didgeridoo

If you can find someone who is playing didgeridoo in your area, that is the ultimate way to experience this primal and magical sound. However, a good alternative is a set of headphones and an authentic Aboriginal player found on the internet. Close your eyes, and allow yourself to be transported into a meditative or trance state. If there is something troubling you, you may wish to set your intention to acknowledge, address, and release deep emotional patterns, allowing them to drift away on the sound. The rhythm of the didgeridoo is an important part of the experience. Try putting a didge track through speakers and allowing yourself to move with the sound, ground your (preferably) bare feet into the floor with each step, and release your primal urge to dance. Let go, and dance like no one is watching!

VITAMIN F

Frequency, Forks

*What we have called matter is energy, whose
vibration has been so lowered as to be perceptible
to the senses. There is no matter.*

ALBERT EINSTEIN

SCIENTIST AND VISIONARY Nicola Tesla spoke about it.
Einstein agreed. Then, science proved it. It is fact that our own
bodies are made up of energy that vibrates at different frequencies. Can sound frequencies affect us? It appears so.

This chapter addresses the carrier wave of sonic vitamins,
frequencies, and their finely crafted instruments, tuning forks.

FREQUENCY

Frequencies affect other frequencies, much like combining
ingredients with other ingredients affects the taste of a meal.
The way frequencies affect the physical world has been demonstrated through many experiments, such as those in the
science of cymatics and water memory. As discussed previously, cymatics provides physical evidence that when sound
frequencies move within a medium such as air, sand, or

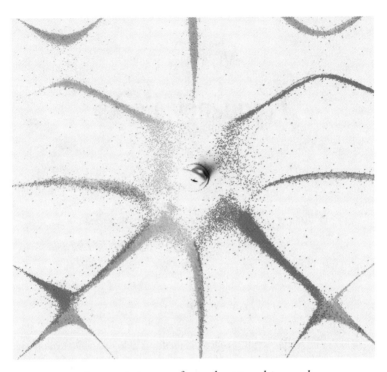

A cymatic image of sound captured in sand

water, they alter the vibration of matter to create amazing patterns.

Memory captured in water illustrates how our intentions can alter the material world. It has been proved by Masaru Emoto, who has conducted studies that show how simple intentions expressed through emotions, thoughts, words, and sound can alter the way water crystallizes. We all hold vibrational frequency, and our bodies are estimated to be about 70 percent water. With so much water to absorb our intentions, it is no wonder that intentions are so powerful in the healing journey. But how do intentions permeate the human body? There is a new scientific theory that we have an "organ" in our body called the mesentery, previously thought to be a few fragmented structures in the digestive system. A recent article in *The Lancet* recognized it as an organ filled with fluids that connect to the lymphatic system and thereafter the whole body.[1] As the power of sound to affect change on water has been demonstrated, it follows that sound will beneficially affect this organ, which is responsible for much of our well-being.

The images shown, taken from the work of Masaru Emoto in his book *The Hidden Messages in Water*, demonstrate the power of sonic words and intention on water molecules. When the words *well done* are applied to water, which is then frozen and a section photographed, the crystal is beautiful to behold. However, when the admonition *you fool* is applied, the result is misshapen and unpleasant. This is why it is so important to monitor how we speak to ourselves. Imagine the impact

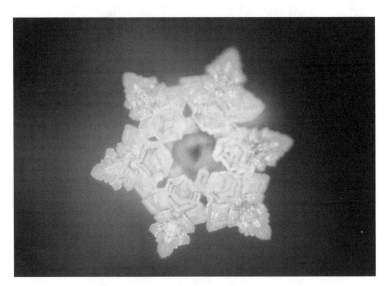

Water's reaction to the words well done.
From Masuru Emoto, The Hidden Messages in Water.
Image courtesy of the Office Masaru Emoto, LLC

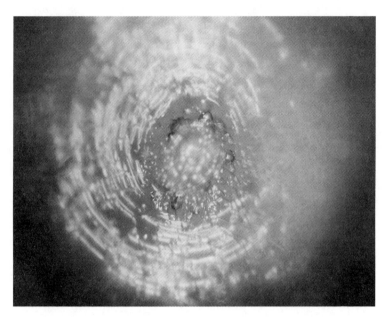

Water's reaction to the words you fool.
From Masuru Emoto, The Hidden Messages in Water.
Image courtesy of the Office Masaru Emoto, LLC

of insulting your body's water reserves! Frequency and intent, whether through thought, voice, sound, or music, have a powerful effect.

It is said that Hitler used sonic mind manipulation. He played extremely low frequency (ELF) radio waves that made the crowds in front of him feel sick or emotionally uneasy because these frequencies disrupt human biorhythms and affect brain waves. If he wanted them to rally against something, he turned these low frequencies up. When he wanted the crowds to be inspired by his words, he turned them off completely. The sense of relief in the physical body and the release from discomfort and, therefore, subsequent emotional uplift could be associated with his words and message.[2]

So, it is demonstrated that music and frequencies can alter our vibrational and, therefore, physical, emotional, and mental states.

In addition to this, sound can kill viruses. In 2008, Russian researchers mathematically determined the frequencies at which simple viruses could be deactivated. This arises from an inherent characteristic of all objects called *resonant frequency:* the frequency at which an object naturally vibrates. Everything has its own resonant frequency. Think of how glass shatters when the perfect note is sounded (often high A). Sound is so powerful it can be used as a military weapon. Equally, that power can be harnessed as an instrument for healing. The most astonishing experiment that was performed by Dr. Pjotr Garjajev's group is the reprogramming of DNA codon sequences using modulated laser light. (Light is frequency at very high speed.) By modulating certain frequencies onto the laser light, they were able to reprogram in vivo DNA in living organisms by using the correct resonant frequencies of DNA. The most impressive discovery made so far is that spoken language can be modulated to the carrier wave with the same reprogramming effect.[3] It follows that our own DNA can simply be reprogrammed by human speech, supposing that the words are modulated on the correct carrier frequencies! Therein lies the power of affirmations, chants, and song.

So, what is frequency? Sound and vibration can be shown in waves and delineated as cycles per second (that is, the number of waves per second). This measurement is also called Hertz (Hz) after the German physicist Heinrich Hertz. A sound event that repeats once per second is 1 Hz.

When we start to look at frequency, we are also taken into the realm of divine mathematics, the blueprint on which all life in the universe is based. Much of our historical knowledge

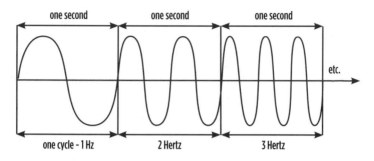

Frequency shown as waves per second.
The more waves per second, the higher the frequency.

about the correlation between divine ratio and music comes from the Greek philosopher and mathematician Pythagoras, who traveled for twenty-one years and studied in Egypt and Babylon, where he learned the mystical and secret association of music and number. Pythagoras calculated the ratio of musical intervals and a system of scales we use today in Western music. To him, music was a primary source of knowledge, and there was no difference between the study of music and the study of how our world works. He was keenly aware of the vital bond between the two.

Mathematics is a complex subject on which many books have been written. For the purpose of this one and from the point of view of sound healing, we will need to understand the golden ratio or phi, the Fibonacci series, and Pythagorean and solfeggio scales.

The golden mean or ratio is the mathematical ratio that can be seen everywhere in nature. It appears in the greatest galaxy and the smallest shell, including the cochlea inside the human ear, which is shaped like a shell. Our very sense of hearing is designed to perfectly match the codes of creation. Our eyes also register this beauty when beholding this ratio in nature, in the

$$\frac{a+b}{a} = \frac{a}{b} = \phi \approx 1.61803$$

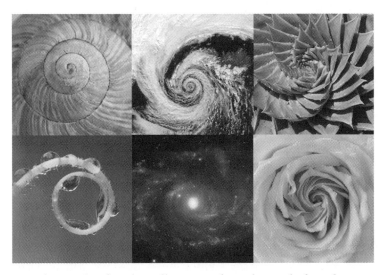

The golden mean expressed in mathematics and symbolically

*The spiral is found in all creation from the swirl of a galaxy
to the curve of a flower's bloom.*

human face, and in great works of art. The spiral also expresses the Fibonacci sequence, named after an Italian mathematician, Leonardo of Pisa, later known as Fibonacci. His sequence maps a predictable and infinite pattern of growth and structure. The Fibonacci sequence is expressed in nature's spiral; branching in trees, the arrangement of leaves on a stem, the fruit sprouts of a pineapple, the flowering of an artichoke, the uncurling of a fern, and the arrangement of a pine cone's bracts. The first two terms in the sequence are the integers one plus one, and each successive term is the sum of the two immediately preceding.

$$1 + 1 = 2$$
$$1 + 2 = 3$$
$$2 + 3 = 5 \ldots \text{and so on into infinity}$$

As we stay with divine numerology, the Book of Revelation, channeled and written on the Greek island of Patmos, talks about a pivotal number of people, 144,000, who would learn to sing a new song that no man would learn except the 144,000 who were redeemed from the Earth. If we apply Pythagoras's theory that all large numbers can be reduced to the sum of the single digits, then the number 144,000 can be reduced to $1 + 4 + 4 = 9$. Nine is the number of completion before a new cycle begins. Divine mathematics, indeed. There are many interpretations and expectations surrounding the Book of Revelation. I tend to believe that the stories are allegorical rather than literal, as if deep knowledge was given to be understood when we are ready. I think it shows that when a critical mass of people raise their vibration, a new age will be born for humanity. Sound healing is all about raising vibration and frequency.

Human Ear Anatomy

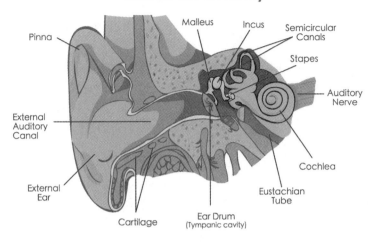

The cochlea shell at the heart of the human ear.
Notice that the structure of the cochlea is a spiral.

FORKS

Tuning forks are exquisitely and finely tuned to carry sound frequencies to activate healing mechanisms in the human body. Some tuning forks are designed to be struck, or activated, then passed in and around the auric field and particularly either side of the head to balance brain hemispheres. Others are weighted and are designed to be placed on the body to send vibration directly into the tissues. These are called osteophonic or Otto tuners, and some have the addition of crystals to amplify their effect. When tuning forks are struck and held on either side of the head, the difference between the frequencies each carries is the binaural beat that synchronizes the right and left hemispheres of the brain. (For example, activating Pythagorean tuning forks with the notes C equal to 256 Hz and G equal to 384 Hz, creates a mathematical interval between them which is called a perfect fifth in music.) Using this interval alone, in thirty seconds (the time it takes to stretch a muscle) you can achieve the same state of deep relaxation that might take thirty minutes to reach with meditation.

If you wish to become a student of intervals and the protocol of using them, John Beaulieu's book *Human Tuning* is a seminal work. There are ranges of Om tuners, crystal tuners, angel tuners, chakra tuners, Fibonacci tuners, solfeggio tuners, and body tuners. A good source of information on tuning forks is Biosonics, the website of John Beaulieu from whom I have learned much of my work with tuning forks. I would also recommend you to my dear friend and mentor, Debbi Walker of Suara Sound, whose courses encompass Om tuners and the solfeggio range plus many frequencies of ancestors, nature, astral bodies, and the divine masculine and feminine.

I have many sequences of tuning forks in my therapy room, each with their own magical purpose. One of the first sequences I used was a series of body tuners based on the fundamental frequency of 8 Hz, which equates to the Schumann Resonance of the planet. As mentioned earlier in the book, this frequency fluctuates, but 8 Hz is a reasonable mean figure. If we take 8 Hz as the base, then double the frequency to 16 Hz, then double the frequency again to 32 Hz, and so on, you see the ratio of these body tuners to the fundamental frequency of the planet we live on.

This seems a good moment to address a tuning that has attracted much publicity in recent years. When an orchestra or solo musician tunes their instrument to "concert pitch," they use a standard tuning: the note A equal to 440 Hz. This standard is relatively recent, set by the International Standards Organization (ISO) in 1953. Many consider that this frequency is too high, or too tight. Looking at the vibratory nature of the universe, it's possible that this pitch is disharmonious with the natural resonance of nature and may generate negative effects on human behavior and consciousness.

When working with sound healing, the preferred tuning is A = 432 Hz. It is said that Beethoven was a fan of 432 Hz tuning. Also, the Stradivarius violin, a very well-known and prized type of violin, works best tuned to 432 Hz. Furthermore, there is a suggestion that music tuned to 432 Hz causes less hearing damage when played at loud volume.[4]

Why is the 432 Hz tuning so desirable? If we return to 8 Hz as the basis for resonance of our planet and therefore naturally in tune with living organisms, the frequencies raised from 8 Hz would also be so. 432 Hz is part of this cycle.

Another instance why 432 Hz might be a beneficial tuning is recorded by the HeartMath Institute in Colorado. Their research reported that the heart's normal frequency is 250 Hz.[5] Now this frequency is quite close to middle C on the piano, roughly 261.6 Hz on a tempered tuning. However, if the piano tuning is adjusted to use A equals 432 Hz, then middle C comes to 256 Hz, even closer to the HeartMath Institute's measurement.

In his time, the visionary Rudolph Steiner proposed that our Western tuning system should be based on A equal to 432 Hz. Proportionally, this tuning would, in turn, make C equal to 256 Hz.[6]

Some theories (although unproven) even suggest that the Nazi regime had been in favor of adopting the higher pitch of 440 Hz as standard after conducting scientific research to determine which range of frequencies best induce fear and aggression. Whether or not this is true, interesting studies have pointed toward the calming benefits of tuning music to A at 432 Hz instead.

This resonance, 432 Hz, is said to be mathematically consistent with the patterns of the universe. It vibrates with the universe's golden mean phi and unifies the properties of light, time, space, matter, gravity, and magnetism with biology, the DNA code, and consciousness. When our atoms and DNA start to flow in harmony with the spiraling pattern of nature, our sense of connection to nature is magnified. The number 432 is reflected in ratios of the diameter of the sun, Earth, and moon, as well as the timing of the precession of the equinoxes, the measurements of the Great Pyramid of Egypt and Stonehenge, and the Sri Yantra mandala, whose 43 interlocking triangles that symbolize the cosmos are mathematically precise and based on the golden mean.

Another interesting fact worth considering is that an A equal to 432 Hz tuning correlates with the chakra system and corresponding color spectrum, while A equal to 440 Hz does not. So, it is not surprising that when the fundamental note of a scale is altered, it no longer corresponds to the color but shifts by approximately one semitone.

The ancients instinctively tuned their instruments at an A of 432 Hz instead of 440 Hz—and for a good reason. There are plenty of music examples on the internet that you can listen to in order to establish the difference for yourself. Tuning instruments to 432 Hz results in a more relaxing sound and state of presence; a 440 Hz tuning may cause you to feel slightly tense.

John Beaulieu, world-renowned sound healer and author of *Human Tuning,* explains:

> The A 432 is based on the Pythagorean spiral. At Biosonics, we encourage and support you to mindfully experiment with different sounds. The best way to under-

stand the effects of sound is to listen and observe how the sound effects your mind and body. Discussions on ideal tuning systems have been going on in every culture for thousands of years. As it turns out there are literally thousands of different ways to tune an instrument, and thousands of different arguments for and against different tuning systems. We would prefer you have the opportunity to directly experience the sound, and then learn about the qualities others ascribe to the sound.[7]

Wise words! Use your own experience. As with so much of life, if something doesn't resonate with you, try another system. As human organisms, we are ever changing. What works for one may not work for another. Or what works one day may not the next. We are not static beings, and our needs change as our vibrations shift. With one client, I may use the Pythagorean body tuners, and for others, I may switch to the solfeggio range.

The solfeggio range of tuners is based on the "rediscovery" of a series of frequencies in a hymn written by eighth-century Lombardian historian Paulus Diocanus. It was the plainchant (Gregorian) hymn to John the Baptist.

Ut queant laxis,
resonare fibris,
mira gestorum,
famuli tuoram,
solve polutti,
labii reatum,
Sancte Johannes.

In the eleventh century, Italian music theorist Guido de Arezzo developed a six-note scale, which will be familiar to modern music students, or anyone who has watched the film *The Sound of Music*. De Arezzo's scale was:

Ut, re, mi, fa, sol, la

Or perhaps more familiarly:

doh, re, mi, fa, sol, la*

The hymn's first six lines of the music commenced respectively on the first six successive notes of the scale, and thus the first syllable of each line was sung to a note one degree higher than the first syllable of the line that preceded it. Because the music held mathematic resonance, the original frequencies were capable of spiritually inspiring mankind to be more "god-kind."

UT *queant laxis*
RE *sonare fibris*
MI *ra gestorum*
FA *mili tuoram*
SOL *ve poluti*
LA *bii reatum*

Rather like the Sanskrit chant *Om Mani Padme Hum*, which we met in Vitamin C, the hymn is difficult to translate and has many layers. However, one broad interpretation is that these six frequencies can assist us in opening up our energy channels to harmonize, balance, and allow the life force energy to flow freely and bring optimum health. A commonly quoted

---

*The syllable *ti* was added later.

literal translation from Latin is: "In order that the slaves might resonate (resound) the miracles (wonders) of your creations with loosened (expanded) vocal cords. Wash the guilt from (our) polluted lips. Saint John." In other words, the hymn was created so that people could peacefully express the miracle of life and God's blessings, thus revealing their true spiritual voice and nature. The translation seems to suggest that solfeggio notes open up a channel of communication with the Divine.

How did the syllables connect to the solfeggio frequencies? In the mid-1970s, Dr. Joseph Puleo, a physician and America's leading herbalist, found six electromagnetic sound frequencies that corresponded to the syllables from the hymn to St. John the Baptist. According to the documentation provided in *Healing Codes for the Biological Apocalypse,* coauthored with Leonard G. Horowitz, Puleo was introduced, through an open vision, to the Pythagorean method of numeral reduction. Using this method, he discovered the pattern of six repeating codes in the Book of Numbers 7: 12–83.

In his book *A Fork in the Road,* David Hulse, a sound therapy pioneer with over fifty years of experience, described the tones as follows:

UT – 396 Hz – turning grief into joy, liberating guilt and fear
RE – 417 Hz – undoing situations and facilitating change
MI – 528 Hz – transformation and miracles, repairing DNA
FA – 639 Hz – relationship, connecting with spiritual family
SOL – 741 Hz – expression and solutions
LA – 852 Hz – awakening intuition[8]

In addition to this original discovery, there are three frequencies that can be calculated below the 396 frequency before breaking the pattern (63, 174, 285) and there are infinite frequencies that can be calculated above the 852 frequency. Many sound healing practitioners use a set of nine tuners that incorporate these extra frequencies. The digits of the solfeggio frequencies as well as the digits of these additional frequencies can be added to produce a sum, the digits of which will be equal to 3, 6, or 9, as shown below:

174: $1 + 7 + 4 = 12$ $1 + 2 = 3$
285: $2 + 8 + 5 = 15$ $1 + 5 = 6$
396: $3 + 9 + 6 = 18$ $1 + 8 = 9$
417: $4 + 1 + 7 = 12$ $1 + 2 = 3$
528: $5 + 2 + 8 = 15$ $1 + 5 = 6$
639: $6 + 3 + 9 = 18$ $1 + 8 = 9$
741: $7 + 4 + 1 = 12$ $1 + 2 = 3$
852: $8 + 5 + 2 = 15$ $1 + 5 = 6$
963: $9 + 6 + 3 = 18$ $1 + 8 = 9$

If you only knew the magnificence of the 3, 6, and 9,
then you would hold a key to the universe.
NIKOLA TESLA, SCIENTIFIC VISIONARY AND
GENIUS OF ELECTROMAGNETIC ENGINEERING

⊙ Ways to Take Vitamin F

Listen to the Frequencies

As we have seen, inside our ears is a shell designed in perfect symmetry with the codes of creation. The universe gifted you this treasure for a purpose, so take the time each day to listen.

- Sit in silence and listen to your body, your heartbeat. With practice, you will be able to hear more, including your nervous system and intuition. Becoming silent is an art, and we are trained from infancy to listen to external cues. However, with meditation and focused attention, you will begin to hear the inner workings of your body (see Vitamin S, silence).

- Listen to music that is recorded using the 432 Hz tuning. There are many examples of Beethoven recorded in this pitch. It is said that John Lennon's *Imagine* was recorded in this tuning. You will find recordings of the solfeggio tones on the internet that you can purchase and download.

- Or listen to a recording of *Ut queant laxis* and intone with it. This is how the original frequencies were used.

- Book a session with a professional sound healer who can bathe you in frequencies from tuning forks, bowls, and voice.

- Or, if you are an accomplished singer, with perfect pitch, you might like to sing the frequencies. You'll both hear the frequencies and experience their vibrations within the body.

Sonic Power and Sleep

Bathe in the sound frequencies while drifting off to sleep. If there is a particular area of your life that you would like to work on, tell your mind to pay particular attention to that frequency as you lay your head on the pillow. Suara Sound offers several CDs based on *Om*. You will also find a wide range of options by Jonathan Goldman. And I have recorded a short fifteen-minute meditation called "Solfeggio Sleep" that you will find on my YouTube channel.

Recommendations about Tuning Forks

You might like to buy your own set of tuning forks. If you are going to do this, it is worth getting the best quality you can as the fine-tuning of the frequency is important. Jonathan Goldman and Biosonics have a good range. Suara Sound offers many based on goddesses and divinities. You should NOT use a weighted Otto tuner above the waist on the chest cavity if you are fitted with a pacemaker. A non-weighted tuner is safe. But always use your common sense. Do not vibrate it close to the chest wall. If you have a pacemaker and experience anything unsettling, please cease immediately.

Gongs

GONGS ARE SOUND HEALING INSTRUMENTS that deserve their own chapter. A gong bath is a form of sound therapy where a single gong, or multiple gongs, are played in a therapeutic way to bring about energetic balance or healing. This can be done individually or as part of a group treatment.

During a gong bath, you are bathed in sound waves. There is no water involved nor clothes removed. Gongs hang in their strong steel frames around the room, and sonic healing is received lying down either on the floor or a couch. Some gongs, like the moon gong, are relatively small—the size of a tea tray—while others, such as the mighty sun gong, are heavyweights and three feet in diameter. Striking or caressing a gong with specially designed mallets creates a sonic sound wave. Because it covers the full spectrum of sound, the gong vibrates all cells, bones, and organs. Depending on the pitch of the gong, you may feel an influx of positive energy in some areas of your body more than others. Experiencing the tone of the gong is referred to as "feeling tone" because one feels it in the body.

It was said by the ancients that if you were bathed in sound waves from a gong for ten days, you would be cured of anything. The current opinion of the scientific community is that the use of sound is becoming an ever more valuable tool in the treatment of many conditions, ailments, and diseases. As an alternative medicine, it is being used successfully all over the world. The corporate world has recently become aware of the therapeutic benefits of gong bathing, and major companies are now booking lunchtime gong baths for their staff.

Gong baths have astounding and wondrous effects on a whole range of maladies. Gong baths can help with physical, mental, or spiritual concerns by bringing about the transition of cellular realignment through the medium of sound. The pure sound waves of the healing gong will enable you to break free of old patterns and regenerate and rebalance yourself as there is nowhere that the resonance of the healing gong cannot penetrate. The healing resonances from the gong will bypass the mind and go straight to the root of the problem.

Gongs come in a variety of sizes and tunings. Most are manufactured and tuned in the Paiste factory in Germany. The Paiste family has been making gongs for generations and has handed down the ancient art of making rich-sounding, melodious gongs to this day. The methods used in manufacturing date from earliest times and consist of individual manual work, which is expensive and time-consuming. But machines could never replace the skill and sacred art of fine-tuning each individual gong, the human touch. Mechanized production of gongs would destroy their spiritual sounds. Each gong has been tuned at the Paiste factory to an exact frequency pitch, or resonance.

Although there are others, you are most likely to encounter planetary gongs, and therefore I will concentrate on these. A symphonic gong has a universal sound structure, and is a convenient gong to own if you have neither the space nor finances to purchase a full planetary set. Planetary frequency was formulated based on the original work of Johannes Kepler in the 1700s, and by Hans Cousto the Swiss scientist whose seminal work *The Cosmic Octave* is the basis for sound healers the world over.

How does a gong sound like a planet? Hans Cousto devised formulas that describe how we are able to hear each planet energetically. The Earth year gong, for instance, is tuned to 136.10 Hz, also the frequency of the central Om tuning fork (see Vitamin F, forks). If you would like to know how such mathematical precision is calculated, the explanation is as follows. An Earth year is broken down into seconds. A day has 86,400 seconds, and a year has 365.2425 days. Multiply the days by the seconds and the answer will be 31,556,952 seconds. Cousto's formula is then applied to arrive at a number that is within two decimal points of the frequency used to create the gong. The frequency for the Earth year gong will be 136.10 Hz, musical note C#. The other planetary frequencies are calculated using our knowledge of their orbits around the sun and their rate of spin. If you are interested in the more formal version of Cousto's science, I strongly suggest you read *The Cosmic Octave*.

Yogi Bhajan, master of kundalini yoga, explains it like this:

> The Gong is the first and last instrument for the human mind, there is only one thing that can supersede and command the human mind, the sound of the Gong. It is the first sound in the universe, the sound that created this universe. It's the basic creative sound. To the mind, the sound of the gong is like a mother and father that gave it birth. The mind has no power to resist a gong that is well played.

Sixth-century BCE Greek philosopher, mathematician, musician, and cosmologist Pythagoras developed the concept of the music of the spheres, the tone of each planet in our solar system coming together as one great cosmic chord. Solar system gongs bring the harmonic convergence of the celestial bodies as pure sound energy.

Named for the Greek gods, the planets also embody significant archetypal, astrological, and mythological associations.

ATTRIBUTES OF THE GONGS OF OUR SOLAR SYSTEM		
1. For Endurance, Strength, or Courage	Sun Gong	126.22 Hz
2. For Communication, Clear Thinking	Mercury Gong	141.27 Hz
3. For Love, Harmony, or to Gain Perspective	Venus Gong	221.23 Hz
4. For Sexuality or Emotional Issues	Moon Gong	210.42 Hz
5. For Relaxation, Opening the Heart	Earth Gong	136.10 Hz
6. For Energy or Assertiveness	Mars Gong	144.72 Hz
7. For Trust or Feelings of Prosperity	Jupiter Gong	183.58 Hz
8. For Understanding or Concentration	Saturn Gong	147.85 Hz
9. For Spontaneity or Fluidity	Uranus Gong	207.36 Hz
10. For Vision or Inspiration	Neptune Gong	211.44 Hz
11. For Integration, Purification, Letting Go	Pluto Gong	140.25 Hz

☾ Ways to Take Vitamin G

Choosing a Gong

Given the eleven planetary gongs and their attributes, how should we select a gong to play, listen to, and meditate with?

* Listen to your intuition, and choose whatever feels right to you. By listening to a gong CD or other quality recording, find the planetary gong sound frequency that resonates most with you.

- Look at the solar system gongs descriptions and keywords, and decide on the areas that you would like to enhance or transform.
- Determine the ruling planet of your astrological sign, or consult your astrological chart.
- Experience a gong bath featuring the complete collection of eleven solar system gongs. You will hear each gong individually and collectively to help you decide which planetary frequencies most resonate with you and your purpose.*
- If you can't find a gong bath session in your area, there are many excellent recordings on the internet. I would recommend listening via headphones if you wish to fully immerse yourself without distraction. Gong bathing is a meditative process, so you might choose to listen as an accompaniment to your daily meditation practice. If you can find the time for a gong bath in the morning, that would be a wonderful way to begin your day. Conversely, a gentle moon gong bath would be soothing at the end of the day. And, when there is a full moon, harness the power of astrology and the gong by listening to the planetary gong associated with the astrological sign of that moon.

For me, the sound of gongs is ethereal, galactic, and quite unlike any other form of sound healing. It is well worth experiencing if you have the opportunity!

---

*To experience a gong bath in person, you will need to find a gong master or sound healer in your area who incorporates gongs in his or her offerings. If you live in the South East region of England, Mark Swan is a gong master who can draw on his knowledge, full set of planetary gongs, and much more. I am indebted to Mark for introducing me to this form of healing, and more information can be found on his website.

Listening, Laughter

There's a lot of difference between listening and hearing.

G. K. Chesterton, writer

HERE WE MEET TWO FORMS of sound healing that can not only improve our health but can also improve our social skills.

LISTENING

As I mentioned in my preface to this book, listening and becoming aware of my reactions formed the beginning of my work with sound. On initial examination, you may not consider listening a sonic vitamin, but let me tell you how I came to understand that it is. Listening, along with silence (Vitamin S), are both essential to our growth and well-being. As we have seen earlier in this book, true silence is extremely rare. Even a state of quiet is becoming a rare commodity in our industrialized and electronics-filled surroundings. Is it any wonder, then, that we have lost the art of listening? And yet, so much can be gained by choosing to turn our attention from the daily clamor of multitudinous sound, and instead tuning in to the voices and sounds that matter. When we settle into this quiet place and listen, creativity and healing can flourish.

 Silence is a state of constant expectation and possibility.

Far from being merely silent, being in a listening state where we are receptive, alert, and aware of what we are receiving is very therapeutic. When we listen with attention, we can become aware of whether we are attuned or not. If you are receiving a healing with an instrument—such as a gong, a tuning fork, a singing bowl, or a voice—far more is achieved by gently placing focus on the sounds being beamed. When we listen, we allow the sounds to interact with us, and we become open to their healing properties. With practice, you can become aware instantly when you are out of tune with a frequency or rhythm.

Listening deeply to music is a wondrous gift. When we immerse ourselves in music, as we would at a concert, the harmony, the lyrics, and the rhythm connect to our emotions. Music can then be an uplifting force as opposed to "muzak" (such as that heard in malls and department stores) in the background.

Listening is more than the opportunity to take in healing sound. It is also the opportunity to listen to others and ourselves. When we really listen, without thought of trying to interject our point of view, we open the door to understanding and offer ourselves the potential to grow emotionally.

Making a conscious decision to listen when another is speaking, especially if we are in discord with them, allows you to be fully present and really hear what they are saying, rather than what you think they are saying. How often in conversation are we mentally rehearsing what we plan to say next, rather than waiting to hear the full exposition of the argument? Listening is a skill that enhances all relationships, even if in the listening we realize that we need to put personal boundaries into place. Perhaps, we ourselves feel we have not been listened to, or perhaps, we have not been clear in making our voice heard.

Another form of listening is listening to our own intuition. If you have a sense that your life is not in balance, or sense not to step into the road, not to go to a certain place, or not to follow a course of action, listen to yourself. As I said in the opening chapters, listening and being open to a wider interpretation of life's choices was my initial path into a life of sound healing.

Cultivate the skill of listening, and the world of sound becomes a treasure trove of understanding and potential for healing.

LAUGHTER

How often have you heard these phrases? Laughter is the best medicine. You need a good laugh! Smile and the world smiles with you.

Charlie Chaplin wrote the music for the final scene of the movie *Modern Times*. Later, John Turner and Geoffrey Parsons added lyrics, and Nat King Cole sang the famous lines:

Smile, though your heart is aching . . .

The comic genius Chaplin understood the power of a smile.

Now, neuroscientists have found that even if we fake a smile when we feel down, the action of coordinating muscles to make a smile causes a chemical reaction in the brain that releases dopamine, a neurotransmitter that causes feelings of happiness. Two scientists at University College London, Andreas Bartels and Semir Zeki, searched for the brain structures responsible for affection, love, and smiling. They used fMRI (functional Magnetic Resonance Imagery) to discover that two brain structures trigger smiling, good will, and cooperation.[1] Inquiring minds might like to know the names of these two structures. The nucleus accumbens is one of the structures, and the ventral tegmental area is the second. These two structures activate the neurotransmitter dopamine, which further produces laughter, smiling, and pleasure. Smiling and laughter have the power to make you feel better, even when you are not feeling at your best, because of the chemical reaction in the brain. The key to happiness is just a smile away. Maintain a fake smile for twenty or more seconds for seven days, and it creates a neural network in your limbic system. Continue for twenty-one consecutive days and fake smiling becomes a neurological habit operating on autopilot as a genuine smile. Smile, right now, and see how you feel. According to the research, apparently, we can't tell the difference when looking at a real and a fake smile. Neither can your body. So smile, and fake it until you make it!

Smiling is also shown to activate the leukocytes (white blood cells), phagocytes, lymphocytes, and macrophages in your bloodstream. Their job is to attack foreign bacteria, viruses, and toxins. Smiling is also an antidote to stress. Prolonged stress, many scientists believe, is a state of disease, which can lead to illness and physical breakdowns. Just smiling can give your body the boost it needs to stay healthy.

If you extend that good humor into laughter, it gets even better. An article in *Yale Scientific Magazine* explains that laughter can increase tolerance to pain, lower blood glucose levels in patients with type 2 diabetes, cause the production of nitric oxide (NO), which then triggers a number of cardio-protective processes, and increase the activity of several critical antibodies and natural killer cells essential in antitumor defense.[2]

Making the sound "ha ha" stimulates the tongue and the upper palate of the mouth. It creates useful connections in the brain. That's the secret to using laughter as an exercise.

☺ Ways to Take Vitamin L

Listen Each Day

Carve out time to listen. While this may happen during a certain time of day, there are also ways to tune in naturally to what is around you.

- Listen to conversations around you.
- Listen to the sound of nature.
- Listen to a favorite song and immerse yourself in how you feel.
- Listen to healing frequencies.
- Listen for moments of silence.
- Record your own affirmations and listen to them. The power of listening to your own voice will double the effect.
- Practice listening with a friend or partner. Each takes the time to talk uninterrupted. Document how you feel when you are truly listened to in a journal.

Fake It 'Til You Make It

Smiling is a powerful habit. As we discovered earlier, a fake smile for twenty or more seconds for seven days creates a neural network in your limbic system, and this practice over twenty-one consecutive days turns your fake smile into a genuine smile. Even if it feels false, force yourself to continue to create new neural pathways. A little work is worth the payoff at the end.

- How often and for how long? Twenty to thirty seconds once a day is all it takes. If you want to progress rapidly, practice fake smiling once before lunch and again after lunch. The secret is creating a short, powerful ritual until it becomes a habit after twenty-one consecutive days.
- Practice smiling at every opportunity. Smile at colleagues and complete strangers. Your smile might make their day. It will certainly improve yours. You may even end up laughing!

Laugh Out Loud

When did you last have a really good laugh, the kind of spontaneous laughter we see in children? We remember how good it feels, but we may have forgotten how to do it. You might laugh softly while watching a funny film or reading a comic. But, do you really laugh out loud these days as you did when you were a child? We need to let go and enjoy ourselves again. It is a lost art. If standing in a room of strangers, or even on your own, making *ho ho ho, he he he,* and *ha ha ha* noises seems ridiculous, you might be short of Vitamin L. If you really can't face trying this exercise out loud, why not warm up by thinking and then whispering these sounds to yourself. Go on. Try it!

Just like that smile, fake it until you make it.

- Start with a silent laugh. This is a great place to start according to laughter guru Thomas Flindt. He explains, "Lean your head back and make a silent laugh. Straighten up and try again using a "hmmmm." I bet you find yourself chuckling. If you tend to take yourself seriously, point your index fingers at yourself and let a laugh go. Get together with friends and try a joint laugh. They may think you're mad, but you'll all laugh at it."[3]

• Just like many other practices, laughter is really beneficial first thing in the morning to set up your day. Fling open your arms while still in your pajamas, take in a deep breath, and laugh.

Laugh with Others

If laughter is the best medicine, how do we take it? There is the practice of laughter yoga (hasya yoga), which involves prolonged voluntary laughter. Laughter yoga is based on the belief that voluntary laughter (like faking that smile) provides the same physiological and psychological benefits as spontaneous laughter. Laughter yoga is done in groups with eye contact, jokes, and playfulness among participants.

• Laughter yoga is as much fun as it sounds! In the UK, you can find details of laughter yoga teachers and therapists on the UnitedMind website, or in the US, visit the Laughter Yoga USA website.

• To really feel the benefit of laughing with others, join a laughter club. You will find plenty online. And if there isn't one in your area, get your friends together and start a laughing group. This is also a great practice to take into the workplace. A lunchtime laughter group gets colleagues together and is wonderful for breaking down barriers. You could even set one up online using applications like Skype or Zoom.

• If you'd like a book to guide your practice, try *Laugh: Everyday Laughter Healing for Greater Happiness and Wellbeing* by Lisa Sturge, who shares ten years of experience teaching laughter workshops.

VITAMIN M

Mantra, Music, Mmm Humming

MANTRA

Mantra is a Sanskrit word that means "that which protects and purifies the mind." More simply, *man* means "mind" and *tra* means "tool." In other words, a mantra is a tool for the mind. The word *mind* is intended to encompass the broadest sense of thoughts and the emotions associated with them. A mantra can also be known as a *japa*.

The sacred sound of the mantra contains "seeds" known as bija syllables in Sanskrit. (There are many that I explore in Vitamin V, vowels.) These syllables, when repeated, take seed in the mind and act as a catalyst for change.

Mantras can be recited vocally or mentally. Whereas chanting eventually requires vocal engagement, a mantra is designed to be spoken internally as much as externally. When expressed inwardly, with just the mind, no note or tone is necessary, just a steady rhythm. This is a useful practice to cultivate as it can be called upon at any time and in any situation to gain a sense of calm, balance, and objectivity, especially if our thoughts and emotions are running away with us.

Mantra can be described as sound forms of the consciousness (or *divine* if you prefer that term). All the major wisdom traditions speak of this. They teach that the power of mantra, if used regularly over time, will take you into clarity and awareness, wholeness, or holistic resonance. Although we are probably most familiar with Sanskrit mantras, sacred words exist in many languages, including Hebrew, Arabic, and other languages. Your own name is a wonderful mantra (see Vitamin N).

Recitation of mantra is sometimes accompanied by the use of a *mala,* a circle of 108 beads with an extra guru bead that is often offset and larger than the rest so the fingers can find it when eyes are closed reciting the mantra. Some malas have a differently shaped bead every twenty-seventh bead to guide where you are in the cycle. A mantra is said for each bead. Fingering the beads while chanting a mantra either silently or vocally helps to keep a steady rhythm and thus control and slow breathing. Why 108 beads? The Sanskrit alphabet has 108 letters. Vedic mathematicians measured the sun's diameter to be 108 times larger than the diameter of the Earth, and they measured the distance between the sun and Earth to be 108 times the sun's diameter. In ancient yogic tradition, there are 108 sacred texts of the Upanishads, 108 sacred holy sites in India, and 108 marma (acupressure-like) points on the body. So, chanting a mantra with a mala not only brings focus but also harnesses the power of sacred geometry and vibrational healing.

When we realize the power that sound has in the universe, then it follows that the practice of reciting a mantra is a wonderful tool for healing when unleashed with intent into our consciousness. Using mantra takes us from the outside world to our inner awareness and deep into the subtle layers of the mind. When we engage with our inner world, rather than contracting as we go within, we can actually experience a vast openness and clarity. Our perception has far more room in this great inner space than in the thought-clogged thoroughfares of our consciousness in daily life.

MUSIC

From recorded chants and singing bowls through classical to rock genres, music is, of course, part of sound healing. Have you ever heard a song that engages you so profoundly that it takes hold of your mind's full attention? By engaging our brain and our attention in the right ways, music is able to activate, sustain, and improve our attention. Beyond the obvious application of listening to music for recreational pleasure, music also impacts our emotions, can be used to enhance memory, and aids in the development and improvement of the brain's neuroplasticity.

The idea that listening to certain music could help the brain was put forward by Dr. Alfred A. Tomatis in his 1991 book, *Pourquoi Mozart?* His work was followed by studies by Rauscher, Shaw, and Ky in 1993 in which they found that listening to Mozart, especially piano, improved spatial reasoning. Their findings were followed by a research study in 1997 by Don Campbell, who coined the phrase the "Mozart Effect."[1]

In the time since these first studies, music and singing have been used to help people who stutter. It was found that when they sang, they no longer stuttered. One reason for this effect is that music is an activity in which you use the right side of the brain, whereas language uses the left brain. So, when you sing music, you're no longer exclusively using your left brain.

There are also stories of people with memory loss who regain their identity when they play music. The film *Ladies in Lavender* was a dramatization of this effect and was echoed in real life by the case of the "piano man." Andreas Grassl, a German man, was found in England in April of 2005. When Grassl was picked up by police on April 7, 2005, he was wandering the streets in Sheerness, Kent, in England, wearing a soaking-wet suit and tie, and he did not answer any questions. Remaining silent, he was presented a pen and paper by Medway Maritime Hospital staff in the hope he would write his name. Instead, he drew a detailed sketch of a grand piano. When they first brought him to a piano, he reportedly played music from various genres nonstop for four hours (ranging from classical music by Tchaikovsky to pop music by The Beatles). He remained unidentified for a long time due to his refusal to speak, communicating instead through drawing and playing the piano.[2] During the four months that passed until he suddenly woke up and revealed his identity, the mysterious story spawned media attention and speculation across the world and he was returned to his family in Germany.

There are also two more documented cases showing the power of music to restore the mind. Henry was in a nursing home where he was inert and unresponsive until music was played over headphones. Then Henry started to sing, and then recalled part of his memory and the songs that influenced his youth. His lucidity remained for a while, even when the music was removed, and he was able to hold a conversation.[3] A second case involved Paul, a seventy-nine-year-old man with Alzheimer's. His son, Nick Harvey, sat him in front of a piano and he was able to recall and play a song he wrote back in 1981.[4]

A 2009 study from Petr Janata at the University of California found that there is a part of the brain that "associates music and memories when we experience emotionally salient episodic memories that are triggered by familiar songs from our personal past."[5] In other words, our own familiar music can reconnect people with deep, meaningful memories from their past, as it did in Henry's case.

Neuroplasticity is the brain's ability to reorganize itself by forming new neural connections throughout life, and it can be greatly affected by the interaction of the harmony of music with the brain. Neuroplasticity allows the neurons (nerve cells) in the brain to compensate for injury and disease and to adjust their activities in response to new situations or to changes in their environment. To further clarify, when our brain is damaged, it can find or create new pathways in order to function properly. It's like getting directions to a location. If a road is closed, or you are stuck in traffic, there is sometimes an alternate route to get to the same place. Music can help map that alternate route in your brain.

A great example of this is shown in the case of Gabrielle Giffords, who experienced a brain injury as the result of a gunshot wound that affected her brain's language center and left her almost unable to speak. Through the use of singing and melodic intonation, she was able to provide new information to her mind to create a reorganization that helped her to make the connections necessary to relearn language.

Music is a pathway to our inner world. It helps us to touch and release our emotions when we find ourselves blocked and unable to express them, the business and method employed by music therapists. Music is also a pathway from a locked inner world; it encourages the release of memory and interaction with the outside world.

Music is a magical key.

MMM HUMMING

The letter *M* is the supreme consonant. Humming *Mmm* is the antidote to anxiety. As *Mmm* is the sound of yourself, humming this sound helps with schizophrenia or hallucinations. The *Mmm* sound represents the essential self or sense of "I," draws you inward to a point of inner peace, and is the opposite of ego. Internationally renowned sound healers Jonathan and Andi Goldman have recently written an entire book on humming titled *The Humming Effect,* in which they explore the science behind the power of humming and the many spiritual and therapeutic effects of this self-administered therapy. It is especially useful if you feel ashamed about your voice and find singing or chanting challenging to try. Ritually, the sound of humming is found at the end of *Om,* in *Amen,* and with many of the other sacred seed syllables (see Vitamin V, vowels). The *Mmm* sound doesn't need a pulse; you can modulate it using the tongue. We even make a humming sound when we make a discovery or find ourselves in agreement with another's statement. It is a life-affirming sound.

☺ Ways to Take Vitamin M

Introduction to Reciting Mantra

When you decide to spend time working with a mantra, preparation will bring great reward.

- Find a quiet place where you will not be disturbed and there is not background noise.
- If you want to be vocal and chant, then you will need free airways. Standing is ideal, or sit with your spine erect to allow the abdomen to expand.
- Center yourself by taking some long, slow breaths and exhaling fully.
- Think about your intention. What do you hope to achieve?
- Before making any vocal sound, focus on the sound you wish to produce. It might be spoken, chanted on one note, or it might be a more complex mantra with a tune. Hear it inside you. Concentrate on your intention and allow it to fill you, pushing away outside interference.

- Start repeating the mantra silently. When you are ready and if you wish to do so, after thirty seconds or so, begin to vocalize—chant—the mantra.

- When you have finished, diminish the mantra until it is spoken internally.

- Finally, release the mantra, rest, and maintain silence for at least a minute. It is preferable to spend double the time in silence at the end than you did in the beginning. When working with vibration and sound, much of the healing takes place once the resonance has died away and the effect is internalized (Vitamin S, silence). This is also true of tuning forks (Vitamin F).

Working with More Complex Mantras

Which mantra to choose? We have already met one of the major and most popular mantras, *Om Mani Padme Hum* under Vitamin C, chanting. If you have found some proficiency in working with breath (Vitamin B) and toning on a single note for chakra tuning (Vitamin C), you may feel it is time to try one of the more complex mantras.

 A mantra is a much more complex concept than a mere chant because it is a tool to unite sound, body, mind, and soul in a deeply philosophical or spiritual experience.

There are a great many mantras to choose from. I have shared three that are among my favorites and hold powerful transformational possibilities. In your preparation, you could choose to dedicate your mantra to a situation in the world. Never think you are too small to make a difference. You are far more powerful than you think.

The Green Tara mantra *Om Tare Tuttare Ture Soha* is used by Tibetans and Buddhists. It is pronounced "Om-TAH-ray-TOO TAH ray-TOO ray-soh HA." (The capitals show where to put the emphasis.)

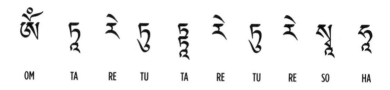

Tibetan script Om Tare Tuttare Ture Soha

The Green Tara mantra brings forth the qualities of compassion in action. The word *Tara* can be translated as "star" or "to cross or traverse." The Green Tara mantra can be used to alleviate physical, mental, or emotional blockages and difficulties in relationships. We need only ask and then release all attachment to the outcome. When we cling to a particular outcome, we create anxiety, agitation, and unhappiness within ourselves. The flow of this mantra relieves clinginess and transports us to peace and clarity.

- Stand, sit, or lie in a comfortable position where you can breathe freely and deeply. Be in silence while you prepare your intention.
- Raise your hands in prayer position in front of your heart.
- Say the mantra in your mind first, and then begin to vocalize it. If you would like to add a simple tune, there are many examples to be found on the internet.

A mantra and healing technique from Hawaii is called *Ho'oponopono*. This ancient Hawaiian phrase is pronounced "ho-oh-pono-pono" and means "I am sorry, Please forgive me, Thank you, I love you."

When I was first introduced to this phrase, I did not use it as a mantra. There may be those who disagree with me that this is a mantra; however, it has long been renowned as a healing phrase. Quickly I realized that it is best used in repetition and makes a good mantra. Furthermore, it is in English for those who are more comfortable speaking their mother tongue. It is one of the most powerful tools for forgiveness and surrender I have encountered, and it works on many levels.

It can be directed toward someone we feel has wronged us. In reciting this phrase, we do not condone his or her actions but instead set ourselves free from constant hurt when we decide to be the one who sees the divinity in another, blesses him or her, and walks away. It is then the responsibility of the other to deal with their own shortcomings. Why would you want to add to your burdens by carrying theirs? Doing so is akin to an excellent saying: "Carrying unforgiveness is like drinking poison and expecting the other person to die."

Equally, the Ho'oponopono phrase can be turned inward to our heart and inner child when we feel we have given away our personal power and allowed ourselves to be manipulated or not behaved as we might have wished. Forgiveness of self or others, making space for healing and gratitude, is one of the most powerful tools we have to release our bonds.

Saying "I love you" opens your heart. Saying "I'm sorry" keeps you humble. Saying "please forgive me" acknowledges your imperfections, and saying "thank you" expresses your gratitude. The mantra will heal your karmic imprint and give you a chance for a fresh start.

In English, the mantra is *I am sorry, please forgive me, thank you, I love you.*

- You can think, say, or chant the four phrases in any order.
- I tend to find myself making a simple three note tune when using it, but, a single note chant will be just as effective.
- Chanting this with 108 beads of a mala would be truly transformative. Also, I have often used it to good purpose while sitting in traffic jams. Why waste time fretting over what we can't control when we can use the time to enrich our lives?

Another more complex mantra is the Gayatri mantra, which is sometimes described as the "mother of all mantras." It is more challenging to learn but well worth the effort. The Gayatri mantra is a six-thousand-year-old verse recited by millions of Hindus every day all over the world. This mantra from the sacred text *Rig Veda Samhita* (3.62.10) was composed by the sage Vishwamitra. One description of its power and influence is that when it is chanted, we enter the quantum field, the place of all possibility beyond time and space—the heart of God. You can tell I'm a fan. It's one of those mantras that makes you feel like you can move mountains.

The mantra consists of twenty-four syllables. It is three lines of eight syllables each. The first line—*Aum Bhur Bhuvaha Swaha*—is considered an invocation and is not technically a part of the original Gayatri mantra as it appears in the Upanishads. It is said to have the most effect when chanted in the morning and evening, which are portals into our day and into our rest and sleep, respectively.

In Sanskrit, the verse is,

> *Aum Bhur Bhuvaha Swaha,*
> *Tat Savitur Varenyam*
> *Bhargo Devasya Dhimahi,*
> *Dhiyo Yo Naha Prachodayat*

As with *Om Mani Padme Hum,* this mantra contains multiple depths. However, a basic translation can be given as,

"Oh God, the Protector, the basis of all life, Who is self-existent, Who is free from all pains and Whose contact frees the soul from all troubles, Who pervades the Universe and sustains all, the Creator and Energizer of the whole Universe, the Giver of happiness, Who is worthy of acceptance, the most excellent, Who is Pure and the Purifier of all, let us embrace that very God, so that He may direct our mental faculties in the right direction."[6] (Capitalization and punctuation in original.)

ॐ भूर्भुव: स्व:

तत्सवितुर्वरेण्यं ।

भर्गो देवस्य धीमहि,

धीयो यो न: प्रचोदयात् ॥

Gayatri mantra in Sanskrit script

The best way to learn the mantra is the method used in ancient times: listening. There are many renditions on the internet that you can use to learn the four phrases. You can chant them on a single note as I did when I studied with my yogi. Or, if you prefer a musical approach, I would refer you to the version by Tim Wheater from his album *Invisible Journeys,* which remains my favorite way to use it. I am indebted to Tim for teaching me this mantra.

Ways to Incorporate Music into Your Life

Immerse yourself in your favorite music. Music helps us release grief when we can't find our way out of that tunnel. Music reconnects us to who we are.

- Mozart and classical music are famous for having a healing effect.
- If classical music does not appeal to you, choose music that you find uplifting. On some days, that might be a lively piece that has you dancing around the room drumming on the table. On other days, it may be a song or piece that brings back happy memories.
- If you play an instrument, allow yourself time to express what you are feeling rather than following a written score.
- If you don't play an instrument, allow yourself to sing something that expresses who you are or how you are feeling.
- If you don't sing, hum!

Humming Your Way to Inner Peace

Everyone can hum. You don't have to be musical. You don't have to sing. Hum happily through your day, and feel your blood pressure lower and your spirits soar. Humming resonates through the whole nasal cavity and vibrates the hard palate at the top of the mouth with its eighty-four meridians. If you want physical proof and a little fun, try humming while holding your nose. You can't. You need access to the whole cavity for the sound to occur.

- To get started, take in a deep belly breath (Vitamin B) and exhale while making the sound *Mmm.*
- Feel your nasal cavity and lips vibrate.
- See if you can direct the sound down your spine to your tailbone so you become a column of sound. After several repetitions, you can round off the practice by extending the hum after saying *Om.*
- If you would like to add a tune, do so.

Nada Yoga, Name, Natural Sounds

NADA YOGA

Nada yoga is the yoga of listening. It is a way to turn inward on a journey that may eventually lead you to enlightenment, but at the very least, nada yoga will fill your daily life with comfort, contentment, and what some call bliss.

BAIRD HERSEY,
THE PRACTICE OF NADA YOGA

Nada yoga is about sounds. It is the journey from everyday sounds to inner peace. It is beyond the scope of this book to go deep into the complexities of nada yoga. However, what follows will introduce you to the origins, philosophy, and the ideas for practice.

Music helps us relax and creates an atmosphere, but nada yoga meditation on the inner sounds reaches profoundly and more precisely into our inner states and has a strong liberating effect in dissolving the very deepest blocks and inhibitions of the mind. Every meditation practice or technique that dissolves the inhibitions of the mind and minimizes its activity is called laya yoga. Therefore, nada yoga belongs under the umbrella of laya yoga. The fifteenth-century saint and mystic poet Kabir described nada like this: "Nada is found within. It is a music without strings which plays in the body. It penetrates the inner and the outer and leads you away from illusion."

The word *nada* comes from the Sanskrit root, *nad,* which means "to sound, roar, or cry." When the letter *a* is added, *nada* means "sound or tone, or to flow like a river." The etymological meaning of *nada* is a process or a stream of consciousness.

Reference to nada yoga can be found in the centuries old *Rig Veda,* a set of Indian verses in Sanskrit. The *Rig Veda* is one of the world's oldest texts.

It is said that nada is the first vibration out of which all creation manifests. And you are a manifestation of that vibration. Just as we are each a unique expression of energy—there is and only ever will be one YOU!—so we all have our note or sound. This is our unique expression of our soul's journey. When you practice nada yoga, your individuality becomes part of the universal consciousness; you become one with it.

Why is it worth practicing nada yoga? Well, for a start, we are all too busy in our heads. We think, we overthink, we fret, and we worry. As an octogenarian of 1910 once said in the *Washington Post,* "Some of the worst things in my life never happened!" If we can turn down the chaos and chatter, peace of mind awaits.

Nada yoga is about how you relate to yourself, how you inhabit your body, how you align your mind, and how you express your soul. It opens a portal to our innermost self, starting with the use of voice and following that sound inward.

It is thought that sound occurs in four dimensions, each denoted by frequency and subtlety or strength.[1] These four levels of sound as taught in nada yoga are *vaikhari, madhyama, pashyanti,* and *para.*

Vaikhari is the everyday sound of the world around us. Some sounds are so familiar we don't notice them. For example, if you tried to sleep in a room with a loudly ticking clock, the sound may keep you awake. However, over time you would become so accustomed to the sound you would no longer hear it. It would become part of the background. We may pay attention to music, alarms, commands, or other sonic cues in our lives, and even sound we no longer hear is present, but ultimately our mind chooses what it will bring to our attention.

Madhyama, the second level of sound, means "between" and is the sound we hear in our mind. Broadly, it is any sound we can imagine or recall. Sometimes these are soothing, like a favorite poem, a loved one's voice, or a piece of music. And other times madhyama is not soothing (think of earworms, those pieces of music that follow us around in our heads). Equally, we can find our mind repeating conversations of criticism or self-recrimination. Madhyama forms the bridge between the world outside and around us and our inner world. Baird Hersey explains that "The same neural pathways within our brains are activated when we recall a sound as were active when we originally heard that sound."[2]

Pashyanti is the third level of sound, the level of sound where the visual world and sounds intersect and eventually merge. For example, consider the experience of listening to sound effects on the radio or a podcast. We create a picture in our mind's eye in response to hearing these effects. We draw on our memory to match images to the sounds. Or we can imagine a visual to match our interpretation of the scene if it is not a situation we have experienced personally. We can listen to music and generate an internal movie. We might extend this to create colors, abstract images, or expressions of what we are feeling in response to sound.

The fourth level of sound is *para,* which means "beyond." Para is accessed when we go deeper, beyond the external world, beyond our sound memories, and beyond our internal imaginings to the still, quiet place inside where there is a sound that is always present within us. It is the vibration of indescribable peace, bliss, or communion with the divine. Para is the hum of the universe.

The Upanishads state clearly about the para sound: "This is Om, this sound is Om."

Nada is sound.
OM is Nada Brahman.
Veda is Nada Brahman.
Sound is vibration.
Name is inseparable from form.
The form may vanish,
but the name or sound remains.
OM is the first vibration of sound.
The world has come out of Nada or OM.
In Pralaya all sounds merge in OM.
Sound vibrations are gross and subtle.
The quality of Akasha [space or ether] is sound.
Akasha is infinite.
So you can fill the ear with the infinite sound.
SWAMI SIVANANDA

NAME

As the teaching in the verses above states, name is inseparable from form. In other words, you came into being and
were named. Your name will endure even when your form has
passed back into spirit. Your name matters; your name gives
you matter. Even the lowliest Tom, Dick, or Harry has a sacred
name.

You may or may not have realized that your name is
sacred. It is sacred because it is *yours*. You may share your
name with other individuals, but nevertheless, the sound
of it is sacred to you. In all likelihood, you chose it. Many
believe that we plant the seed of our name in our parents'
minds while we are still in the womb. You will have heard
the vibration of it as they discussed it, even if that was after
your birth. And from then on, you hear it all your growing
years. The syllables, vowels, and consonants are yours. In
some African cultures, babies are sung into the world using
their name.

Group chanting of your name is a form of sound healing
that is a joy to experience and very powerful. I was first introduced to this in a workshop with musician Tim Wheater. The
recipient was seated in the center of the group. Tim began
with a gentle, rising, three note *Ooooo,* which then changed
into the recipient's name. Some in the circle had instruments
of sound healing, such as singing bowls, wah-wah bars, and
drums. They began to join in the chanting of the name, and
this continued for three to five minutes. Without exception,
those being serenaded reported feeling deeply moved and
blissful. With or without any instrumental addition, this is
a simple and powerful way to invoke a feeling of peace and
being loved.

Another way of doing this is, if the person in the center of the circle receiving the healing knows their fundamental note (see Vitamin V, voice), then the chanters can use that tone. If the receiver's fundamental note is not known, then a designated leader of the circle chooses a tone and orchestrates the beginning and the end of the session. Chanting can be fast or slow (I find slow is preferable), and the orchestrator indicates when to move from one syllable to the next. For example, if the recipient is called Shannon, there are two syllables. If the recipient is named Valerie, there are three syllables to chant.

And finally, using the advances of modern technology, there is a method of using the name in which recipients record their own voice saying their own name (thus guaranteeing a sympathetic frequency and resonance). Then that recording is diminished in frequency by half and augmented by doubling and then doubled again, and the whole is played back during the healing session. There are some specially designed vibro-acoustic sound beds that can play the sound of your name at varying frequencies.

NATURAL SOUNDS

It is documented that the first sense we develop in the womb is hearing, which is also said to be the last sense to go as we leave this world. We are primed by the sounds we hear, and as soon as we emerge, we start making our own. We express our joy, pain, frustration, and needs in a series of cries, tones, gurgles, and giggles. We yawn, we sneeze, and we belch. We release tension from our bodies by making sound, an infantile form of self-healing.

As babies, when we start playing with language, we seem

to talk gibberish. But this is our natural sound and may well be a form of sound therapy for all we know. In some Indian ashrams, there is a practice of talking gibberish to get out of our contained world.

When we yawn, the rush of air—oxygen, prana, or chi (life force)—into our body is revitalizing. Yawning also requires us to open the throat into the *ah* sound, which is connected to the heart chakra.

And of course, there is laughter. It has long been said that laughter is the best medicine (Vitamin L). The key to laughter lies in the hard *H* sound, or *huh*. Although there are many frequencies and vowels in laughter, it is the initial hard *H* sound that gives laughter its healing properties. The power required to expel air to aspirate the *H* works the diaphragm and the chakras. Many a wind instrument player has experimented with producing vibrato by contracting the diaphragm in repeated short *huh, huh, huh* sounds.

At the other end of the emotional scale, we have the natural sounds of groaning and keening. We groan when we are frustrated or in pain. Keening is another word for wailing, the sound of sorrow. So often we are expected to suffer in silence whereas ancient cultures understood the power of expressing emotion to aid us through life's challenges.

And finally, we have sighing and humming (Vitamin M). Sighing is a great release. When we have been afraid or stressed and that situation is over, we sigh with relief. Sighing requires us to take a deep breath and then release. Our shoulders drop the tension and the burden. Humming (Vitamin M) is a comforting sound. We hum when we are happy. A mother hums to her baby. We hum to ourselves. It is a sound that takes us inside to a place of contentment. Both sounds are life affirming and healing, as are all natural sounds.

⊙ Ways to Take Vitamin N

Experience the Power of Nada Yoga

Nada yoga is a journey, and as with all journeys, there are first steps.

- If you wish to work with the power of inner sound, it would be advisable to find a teacher of nada yoga, as this practice is a profound and complex journey.
- If this is not possible, *The Practice of Nada Yoga* by Baird Hersey contains excellent instructions for home-practice techniques.
- Another way to experience inner sound is to visit an anechoic chamber where all external sound is blocked (see Vitamin S, silence). However, it is worth saying that this can be an unnerving experience when first attempted and is best kept to a short, ten-minute session in the beginning. As with all experiences, you are your own best guide to what is acceptable and what feels safe.

Explore the Sonic Qualities of Your Name

If you wish to work with your name, the choices are multiple.

- Try looking at your face in a mirror and addressing yourself by name. You can marry this with a positive affirmation (Vitamin A).
- If you belong to a chanting circle, you could ask to work with your name while you sit in the center of the circle.
- If you know a sound healer who can create personalized recordings, you could request a sonic rendition of your name that can be accompanied by singing bowls or any other heal-

ing sounds imbued with intention to address your concerns. I offer this service via my website, angelhandsheal.co.uk.

Express Natural Sounds

Give yourself permission to make natural sounds. Don't let anyone shame you about your voice, and especially don't shame yourself!

- Hum or sing if you are happy. This is not about entertainment; this is about accessing your right to joy.
- Equally, if you are upset, allow yourself to shout, cry, groan, or even wail. Ideally this would happen spontaneously; however, given the constraints of modern society, you may feel you have to wait for time or space alone. Whichever is the case, do not deny yourself the power and release of voicing natural healing sound.

VITAMIN O

Om

WHENEVER A LAYPERSON THINKS OF CHANTING, it's a fair bet they first think of *Om*. *Om* is the sound of creation. It is said to contain the universe and to have created it. It is the first sound from the beginning of time. When you meditate with or chant *Om,* you are opening a direct portal to the divine and connecting with the whole universal consciousness.

Om is, in fact, a syllable mantra, or Shakti bija mantra. Among the five best-known Shakti mantras, *Om* is called the energy of sound. *Om* serves to open and clear the mind for meditation. It draws the sound current up the spine, through the chakras, and out of the top of the head. It is said to mean "yes"; it is the sound of assent, our agreement to attune to higher realms.

In the beginning was the word, and the word was *Om*. All the major wisdom traditions of the world have a similar text. The Australian Aborigines believe that the world was sung into being. Western science talks of the Big Bang. In the 1950s, space scientists identified a "hum" that they found to be the remaining resonance of the original "big bang," the sound or word that made manifest the universe. Called cosmic microwave background, it remains and continues to underlie our existence.[1] They describe it as sounding like the hum of *Om*.

Om is the ultimate sacred syllable (or more correctly three syllables, as we shall see later). *Om* is a vibrational expression not just on this planet, in this solar system, in this galaxy, throughout this universe, but in *all* creation: the All, the Divine, God, Allah, Jehovah, Brahman, Elohim, to mention just a few (and that's without taking into account the 101 names from Zoroastrianism). Whatever your concept of the great creative force that gave birth to and permeates every living thing in the universe, we are ineluctably linked by vibration.

The ancients knew this. How? Well, we cannot know for sure, but most likely they intuitively tuned in to our planet and the other heavenly bodies. Mathematician and philosopher Pythagoras spoke of the music of the spheres. Now, science can confirm what they knew and recorded in ancient texts. Recently, there was much excitement in the scientific community surrounding the collision of two black holes recorded sending ripples called gravitational waves through the space-time fabric. Perhaps this was a form of rebirth or a reboot of the cosmic blueprint? Time and experience will tell. Our own sun has been recorded by NASA emitting a vibration too low for our human ears that, when adjusted, has been interpreted by some to sound like a hum distinctly close to *Om*.[2]

This sacred syllable is written as *Om*. It is usually recognized in the Sanskrit form, but can also be expressed in the Tibetan form or in Balinese.

There are other expressions, but these three are the most common.

There is some debate whether the mantra is *Om* or *Aum*. The way I like to explain the difference between *Om* and *Aum* is: *Om* is the name of the sound, and *Aum* is how it sounds. This is similar to the various ways of pronouncing the letter *A*.

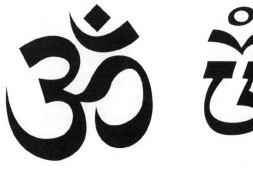

Om *in Sanskrit form*

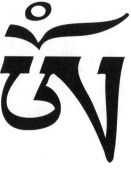

Om *in Tibetan*
Illustration by IFA

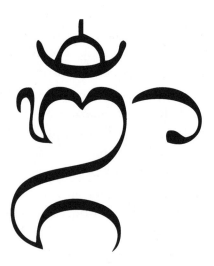

Om *in Balinese*
Illustration by IFA

For example, we say its name as a long *A* as in *hay* but the sound it makes is a short *A* as in *cat*.

Another perspective is that *Aum* is an elongated sounding of *Om,* thus carrying greater opportunity to expand into higher consciousness and allowing the flexibility of emphasis on each syllable. When sounded, *Aum* has three syllables: *Ah, Oo,* and *Mm.* Opinions vary on how to combine them. I have worked with "ah-oo-mm" and "ah-oh-mm." In fact, both options sound very similar when run fluently into each other. Personally, I prefer the first example. *Ah* is the sound of the heart (see Vitamin V, vowels). *Oo* takes me to the bridge between the physical world and the spiritual. *Mm* invokes the power of humming as it resonates in the nasal cavity and vibrates the third eye and crown chakras. It also affects the palatal points of stimuli, the eighty-four nadis in the roof of the mouth.

Om is the center and basis of all that exists expressed in sonic resonance. The central Om tuner in my Om tuning fork set vibrates to the frequency 136.1 Hz, which is also the frequency of the Earth year gong, which is the gong of the heart (see Vitamin G).

☉ Ways to Take Vitamin O

Om is a very versatile vitamin in that it can be absorbed silently or vocally. It can be used to prepare for other sonic vitamins. For example, you could chant *Om* to bring yourself into a calm space before meditation or using an affirmation (Vitamin A). You can vocally chant *Om* (Vitamin C) and use your hands to direct the sound around your aura. It is also a great way to release the debris of the day before you settle down to sleep.

Om and Tuning Forks

If you have an Om tuning fork, start your day by activating the fork and alternately listening to it in each ear three times (as described below), followed by brushing down your aura so that you begin the day fresh and focused. One way to amplify a silent meditation with *Om* is to use an Om tuning fork, either a weighted Otto tuner placed on the breastbone at the center of the heart chakra or a non-weighted standard Om tuning fork that is designed to be heard. (Please do not use a weighted Otto tuner if you are fitted with a pacemaker.)

- If using a non-weighted standard Om tuner, strike it and caress your head by taking the tuning fork from one ear to the other via the forehead, third eye, and over the crown. Allow the body to attune to the sound, take it inside, and meditate on it, hearing the vibration at your core.

- Alternatively, strike the tuner and hold it to your left ear, placing your attention on the sound until you can no longer hear or feel it. Repeat with the other ear. Repeat this for both ears three times. You can continue for ten minutes, and then sit in silence to see what comes.

Om and Chanting

Vocally, *Om* can be chanted by focusing on all three syllables.

- Be aware of the sensations in your body and particularly your chakras as you chant.

- Pay attention to your throat, taking care to keep it open to make the vowels as rounded and resonant as possible.

- In the final stages, close your lips to contain the sound, and feel the buzz of the vibration in your nasal cavity and upper palate, engaging the power of the hum.

- Except for at the close of the chant, each syllable is usually sounded equally. However, if you wish to work on a specific aspect or area of life—for example, heart healing or opening—then emphasis is placed on that syllable.

  - In the case of heart work, give two-thirds of the time to

sounding the first syllable, *Ah,* before flowing through the other two.

- If you wish to work on inner strength, then place more emphasis on the syllable *Oh* or *Oo,* enclosing the sound more quickly at the last moment in *Mm.*
- If you feel the need to resonate the higher chakras and the third eye, then slide the first two syllables quickly to *Mm,* enclosing the sound and maintaining the vibration.

VITAMIN S

~~~~~~~~~~~~~~~~

Silence

Silence is God's first language.
<div style="text-align:right">

SIXTEENTH-CENTURY MYSTIC
ST. JOHN OF THE CROSS
</div>

Everything else is a poor translation.
<div style="text-align:right">

CATHOLIC MONK THOMAS KEATING
REFLECTING ON ST. JOHN
OF THE CROSS'S WORDS
</div>

IN 2011, A WORLD HEALTH ORGANIZATION report called noise pollution a modern plague and concluded that "there is overwhelming evidence that exposure to environmental noise has adverse effects on the health of the population."[1]

We're constantly filling our ears with noise, TV and radio news, podcasts, and, of course, the multitude of sounds that we create nonstop in our own heads. Think about it: How many moments each day do you spend in total silence? The answer is probably very few.

The nineteenth-century British nurse and social activist Florence Nightingale once wrote, "unnecessary noise is the most cruel absence of care that can be inflicted on either the sick or the well." Nightingale argued that needless sounds could cause distress, sleep loss, and alarm for recovering patients.

Decades later, research has shown noise can lead to high blood pressure and heart attacks as well as impaired hearing and decreased overall health. Loud noises raise stress levels by activating the brain's amygdala and causing the release of the stress hormone cortisol.

Just as too much noise can cause stress and tension, research has found that silence has the opposite effect and releases tension in the brain and body.

A 2006 study published in the journal *Heart* found two minutes of silence to be more relaxing than listening to relaxing music and noted that two minutes of silence caused changes in blood pressure and blood circulation in the brain.[2]

Even ten minutes a day, spent in silence, can help you feel less stressed and more focused and creative.

How can silence do this?

According to attention restoration theory, the brain can restore its finite cognitive resources when we're in environments with lower levels of sensory input than usual. In silence—for instance, the quiet stillness you find when walking alone in nature—the brain can let down its sensory guard, so to speak.

Using brain images of people listening to short symphonies by an obscure eighteenth-century composer, a research team from the Stanford University School of Medicine investigated the power between music and the mind and showed that peak brain activity occurred during a short period of silence between musical movements—when seemingly nothing was happening. This led the researchers to theorize that listening to music could help the brain to anticipate events and hold greater attention, just as the listeners demonstrated when they seemed to pay closest attention during the anticipatory silences between musical movements.[3]

In other words: silence sharpens our focus.

The theory is that silence is indeed part of each composer's intention to guide the listener in interpreting the music in his or her brain. It is the space between the notes that captivates our full attention and allows the busy mind to communicate and become congruent with the heart. It is in these silences where our focus is total.

If you ask a musician, composer, or jazz improvisator, he or she will tell you that the gaps between the notes are as important as the notes themselves. Constantly playing without musical pause creates cacophony.

Another benefit of silence is that it can quite literally grow the brain. In 2013, the journal *Brain, Structure, and Function* published research comparing the effects of ambient noise, white noise, pup calls, and silence on rodent brains. Although the researchers intended to use silence as a control in the study, they found that two hours of silence daily led to the development of new cells in the hippocampus, a region of the brain associated with learning, memory, and emotion. While preliminary, the findings suggested that silence could be therapeutic for conditions such as depression and Alzheimer's, which are associated with decreased rates of neuron regeneration in the hippocampus.[4]

Those are the scientific and physical effects. What else can silence achieve?

Creating a regular practice of sitting in silence carries great benefit to our health and mental well-being. We come to realize how much we talk and yet how little is said. Getting acquainted with silence cultivates a mindful use of language and clarity of expression. It also teaches us the art of careful listening. When we really listen to what is said and listen to understand rather than to reply, our communication skills improve. We say what we mean and mean what we say.

⑨ Ways to Take Vitamin S

Complete silence in this world is as rare as hens' teeth. In fact, the only certainty of experiencing it is by sitting in an anechoic chamber. An anechoic chamber is "an-echoic," meaning it is non-reflective, nonechoing, or echo free. It is a room designed to completely absorb even the reflections of either sound or electromagnetic waves, creating a chamber with an amazing amount of absolute nothingness. Absolute silence is filled by the sound of your own body.

Where is the quietest room in the world? For many years, until 2015, Orfield Laboratories in Minneapolis, Minnesota, held the claim. There, scientists had been studying how subjects reacted in their anechoic chamber, also known as the world's quietest room. The sound level in the room, which actually held the Guinness World Record, is negative 9 decibels (compare this to the average "quiet" room's 30). The record is now held by Microsoft's anechoic chamber, measuring a staggering negative 20.35 decibels.[5]

What is usually experienced when a person sits in an anechoic chamber are two sounds: one high pitched and one low pitched. The high-pitched sound is the sound of the person's nervous system, and the low-pitched sound is the person's blood in circulation and often the sound of the beating heart. Given the lack of other sensory input, these sounds can give rise to a more profound physical feeling of the blood pumping through veins.

As most of us are unlikely to experience an anechoic chamber, there are plenty of other ways to cultivate a silent environment.

- Use inexpensive ear defenders to make a place in your home silent so that you can experience your inner sounds.

- Create silence out in nature, where birdsong and gentle leaf rustle serve as the background to quiet contemplation. Sit with your eyes closed and listen. With regular practice, you will attune to nature and recognize a change in the sound of the wind or the symphony of nature and return to the sensitivity our ancient ancestors possessed and wild creatures still do.

- If you are away from home and wish to experience silent moments to achieve peace and balance, closing your eyes and putting focus and gentle attention on the inhalation and exhalation of breath or mentally repeating a mantra are good ways to quieten the mind's chatter to create a peaceful space. To take your attention to your breath, place your focus on the tip of your nose. Feel the sensation of the cool breath entering on the inhale, and the warmer breath leaving on the exhale. Consciously breathe deep into the belly intending to slow the inhale and exhale, each to the count of eight. Initially, if you can't manage eight try four, and progress from there. The actual number doesn't matter; the exercise is to slow the breathing rate. Once the breathing rate is slower, use a mantra with two words, such as *So Ham* (recall the pronunciation "soh-hum"). As your mind travels from the *So* to the *Ham*, pause between the two words and rest in the silence. This takes practice but can yield great results, taking you into a space of inner silence that we rarely have time to experience in our daily lives.

- Strike a singing bowl, and listen to the note die away until you are left contemplating the silence.

- Silence is a wonderful tool when we are facing difficult times in our life. Sit in silence and allow whatever thoughts, sensations, and feelings to arise. So often when challenged, we distract ourselves with retail therapy, drugs, alcohol, food, television, or other modern inventions in the hope that our struggle will all go away. It rarely does! When we cease trying to negate our feelings with worldly distractions and have the courage to sit with our difficulties in silence, we create space to communicate with our truth and find a way to make peace with what is happening. Only then can we release our burdens. Courage is often not the facing of external dangers but the facing of our inner selves and our truths.

- Sitting in silence is a great place to find gratitude. Gratitude is one of the great gifts and powers of human existence, along with forgiveness, which can also be found in the power of silence. Deepak Chopra says: "when you find your gratitude, you find your grace."

Use one of the above methods to sit in silence once a week (or more!), and see how your perception of life changes. You may experience the little daily joys of life more readily, and when storms come, you will weather them better.

VITAMIN V

~~~~~~

Voice, Vowels, Volume

VOICE

For it is only by awakening your heart, by experiencing how it entrains the whole of your consciousness, remembering that it holds within its very centre your divine blueprint, that you may speak the utter truth of your liberation.

THE HEART'S NOTE, STEWART PEARCE

Each voice represents a unique personality that defines an individual's character. Each of us has our unique resonance, our understanding of love, our signature note. Your voice is your most powerful tool—so speak up and speak out!

Your voice is a unique expression of you and a powerful tool for creating vibration and healing. Your voice is your greatest healing instrument. Your voice empowers affirmations, sings, chants mantras, and intones the mighty power of vowels as we will find out later in this chapter.

When we speak, our voice resonates throughout our bodies. We hear ourselves uniquely. It is for this reason we are often surprised when we hear a recording of our voice. Often, we exclaim, "Do I really sound like that?"

Given the power of voice, it is advisable to use this wonderful potential wisely. Think about what you say. Intention is key. In fact, intention + sound = holistic resonance (healing). This equation applies to all sound healing, which is why in previous chapters I have spoken about the importance of preparing mentally before making sound. However, it is particularly pertinent when using your voice, whether to sing, chant, or speak. If we cast back to the first vitamin in this book, Vitamin A (Affirmations), the force of thought coupled with vocal resonance has the power to transform life. Turn to page 137 for an exercise to help you analyze the words you speak and think.

VOWELS

Vowels are like vegetables; they are very good for us. In fact, vowels are so powerful that they were once considered sacred. In ancient written languages, they were often omitted and were reserved for use by the priesthood. The Semitic languages of the Near East, which include Hebrew, Arabic, and Aramaic (the language of the original Lord's Prayer), are written without vowels. If you think this would be impractical, try to read the following:

Hv y vr wndrd bt vwls?

Or should I say: "Have you ever wondered about vowels?" Did you have a problem reading that sentence? You might not have, because our brain has a remarkable ability to fill in the gaps, but vowels certainly make reading easier.

The power of vowels is also linked to the use of breath (see Vitamin B). Breath is our life force. Think about how you say a consonant. Are you able to sustain it? While you can sustain some consonants, like *F, L, M,* or *S,* to sustain the majority of consonant sounds, you need a vowel. Try saying the following words while lengthening their vowels: *teeeeee, boooo, caaaar.* The longer sounds in language are the vowels. Without them, linguistic expression would be limited and lack emotion (because vowels come from the soul of the divine, which is why they were considered sacred). Often the elongation of a vowel for an extended period is referred to as *toning.* Toning vowel sounds is an easily learned skill. All of us have the ability to create pure tone and vocal harmonics. When we first learn to speak, we have a wide vocal range, but as we grow older, our voice begins to become more restricted and closed. Toning oxygenates the body, deepens breathing, relaxes muscles, and stimulates the whole body.

Regular vowel toning helps to restore health to the mind, body, and spirit. Vowel toning will give us a feeling of connection, especially when done with other people. Did you know that when wolves howl (tone), each member of the pack has his or her individual note? As pups in the pack, they listen to the elders and find their own pitch.

Vowel toning strengthens the vocal muscles. It assists in improving our breathing and posture. The muscles of the digestive system are massaged and stimulated by regular toning. Vowel toning can relax and energize us at the same time and can help us to release stress and repressed emotions.

The human voice has a vast potential for healing. Research suggests that toning has a neurochemical effect on the body, boosting the immune system and causing the release of endorphins in the brain. Toning can release psychological stress before surgery, lower the blood pressure and respiratory rate of cardiac patients, and it can also reduce tension in those undergoing MRI and CAT scans. Toning has also been effective in relieving insomnia and other sleep disorders.[1]

And what do we tone? Well, vowels, of course, and humans have done so for centuries.

Pythagoras taught that the human soul, just as the whole world, is created according to musical laws and should be tempered accordingly. In keeping with this, it was said that Pythagoras used to cure people with sound and music. As Diogenes Laërtius wrote in the third century CE, "he used to practice divination by sound or voices." The tradition of chanting vowels is still preserved by Rosicrucians who chant sacred vowels in a certain order and Kabbalists who engage in sound meditation connected with the Sefirot Tree (the tradition that stems from Rabbi Ibrahim Abulafia of the thirteenth century). They believe that this practice harmonizes different levels of their being. So, the tradition of chanting vowels is very ancient. Melanie Braun explains that in ancient Egypt, the laws of music were even engraved on temple walls, vowels from the Oriental languages were used as musical characters, and "invocations to the seven planets were composed of vowels and designated musical modes."[2]

Ancient secrets of sound can also be found encoded in the remarkable mystic carvings in the Lady Chapel arch in Rosslyn Chapel just outside Edinburgh. For many years, they were thought to be merely decorative. Then father and son Thomas and Stuart Mitchel, both musicians, realized that the lines and dots may be cymatic symbols. It took many years of painstaking work to transcribe what was represented into a modern musical stave. The musical piece *The Rosslyn Motet* is now known and available on CD.[3]

Chanting specific vowels can have physiological benefits and also helps with spiritual or personal growth and emotional intelligence.

VOLUME

Sounds in nature, even if loud like a waterfall or roaring ocean, are considered more soothing than sounds of modern life, like traffic.

In fact, sounds over a certain volume go beyond being unpleasant; they can become dangerous. At around 90 decibels, sound becomes damaging. Prolonged exposure at this level can cause hearing loss. Pain begins at around 125 decibels. Loud sound produces a fight-or-flight response that elevates stress hormones and causes the heart rate to accelerate, feelings of irritability or anxiety, and an inability to rest or sleep.

Psychologist Ellen Poliakov of the University of Manchester has studied how sound even affects the taste of food. In her study, participants consumed sweet and salty foods. Subjects wore headphones and tasted food while surrounded by silence, by quiet white noise at 45–50 decibels, and then by louder white noise at 80–90 decibels. They rated the foods less sweet or salty when noise levels were high. This may explain why airline food tastes bland, as average sound in the cabin of a plane can be as high as 80 decibels.[4]

We describe unwelcome volume as "noise."

There are health consequences that follow from regular exposure to consistent elevated sound levels. Elevated workplace or environmental noise can cause hearing impairment, hypertension, ischemic heart disease, annoyance, and sleep disturbance. Changes in the immune system and birth defects have been also attributed to noise exposure. Although some presbycusis, or age-related hearing loss, may occur naturally with age, in many developed nations the cumulative impact of noise is sufficient to impair the hearing of a large fraction of the population over the course of a lifetime. Noise exposure also has been known to induce tinnitus, hypertension, vaso-constriction, and other adverse cardiovascular effects.[5]

Beyond these effects, elevated noise levels can create stress, increase workplace accident rates, and stimulate aggression and other antisocial behaviors. The most significant causes are vehicle and aircraft noise, prolonged exposure to loud music, and industrial noise. In Norway in 2001, road traffic was demonstrated to cause 73 percent of the noise annoyances reported, and coupled with railway and air traffic noise this rose to almost 80 percent of noise annoyance reported.[6]

There may be psychological impacts of noise as well. Firecrackers may upset domestic and wild animals or noise-traumatized individuals. The most common noise-traumatized persons are those who have been exposed to military conflicts, but loud groups of people can often trigger complaints about noise as well as and other behavior-related reactions. Infants are also easily startled by noise.

A European study found that social costs of traffic noise were more than 40 billion euros per year, and passenger cars and lorries (trucks) were responsible for the bulk of costs. Traffic noise alone is harming the health of almost one in every three people in the World Health Organization European Region. One in five Europeans is regularly exposed to sound levels at night that could significantly damage health.[7]

Noise that is outside our control can be tiresome and debilitating. Conversely, sound we make for ourselves can be therapeutic as a vitamin.

☉ Ways to Take Vitamin V

The Power of Words

Develop a habit of monitoring what you say. Perhaps keep a notebook for a week, and write down examples of the way you express yourself. Are you using negative phrases such as: "kill two birds with one stone," "I don't believe it," or "that never works for me"? Why would you want to kill two birds? Instead, you might say: "let's make the most of this possibility!" If you tend to say "I don't believe it" when you have a stroke of luck, you are actually pushing the gift away when you could react with: "I'm delighted it's my turn to be lucky!" What about your use of the superlatives never and always? "I never win." "That always happens to me." Is that really true? You are reinforcing a belief of worthlessness. Worse, you are empowering it with your own voice.

Once you decide to change and begin to monitor your words, you will be surprised how quickly you can turn things around. When you speak words of positive intent, your body and the whole world around you interact with your uplifted vibration. Don't take my word for it. Try it!

Ahhhh . . . That's Better! A Powerful Vowel

Vowels are at our immediate and everyday disposal. The unique benefits of each vowel are described on page 141, but by far the best-known vowel is AH. When we see something we like, we sigh: *Ahhhh*. When we release the burdens of the day, we raise our shoulders then drop them while intoning *Ahhhh*. AH is the sound of our heart, and coincidentally the vowel at the center of the word *heart*. It is also found in many divine descriptions: Amen (AHmen), Allah (AHlah), Jehovah (JehovAH), Brahma (BrAHma), and Krishna (KrishnAH). In order to make this vowel sound, we have to open the back of the throat, thus allowing the free flow of breath.

If you only have time in your day to work with one vowel, the vowel AH offers the greatest power to calm and transform.

- For a really quick treatment when you are stressed, take in a deep breath, down to the belly, and allow the shoulders to rise.

- Drop the shoulders, release the breath, and vocally sigh *ahhh*.
- Repeat three times. How do you feel now?

Vowel Chanting and Toning

Vowel chanting is also a powerful tool. There are various systems for matching chants and vowels to the chakras. The two most common are shown in the tables below.

CHAKRAS MATCHED WITH VOWELS

Chakra	Vowel	Pronunciation
Root	UH	"uh" as in tug
Sacral	OO	"oo" as in zoom
Solar Plexus	OH	"oh" as in Rome but slightly soften to "aw" as in raw. Feel the difference as the back of the throat opens.
Heart	AH	"ah" as in heart
Throat	AYE	"aye" as in say
Brow or Third Eye	EYE	"eye" as in I
Crown	EEE	"eee" as in see

CHAKRAS MATCHED WITH CHANTS

Chakra	Chant (Sanskrit)	Pronunciation
Root	LAM	"l-uh-m"
Sacral	VAM	"w-oo-m" as in book
Solar Plexus	RAM	"r-uh-m"
Heart	YAM	"y-ah-m" as in heart
Throat	HAM	"h-ah-m" (aspirate the *H*)
Brow or Third Eye	OM	"ah-oo-mm" or "ah-oh-mm"
Crown	NG	closed nasal sound "ng" as in hung

I have sat in many circles and heard variations on both of the above systems. The chants in the second table are in ancient Sanskrit. The first table of vowels is a relatively recent innovation. There are other systems based on the harmonic overtones of the human voice that use those vowels in a different order. Please do not get too enmeshed in "performing the right way" or using "the right system." Intention is key, and all chanting is beneficial. This is about entrainment not entertainment or performance.

- To intone the vowels in the first table, begin by choosing a tone in the lower to middle range of your voice, and use that single tone. Once you are confident with that, if you can find the note C, start on the root chakra and work upward. Ideally, you move up a musical tone with each vowel as you work up the chakras. If that is too complicated to begin with, and I am a great advocate of keeping things simple, then use the same note for each chakra and just change the vowel. The benefit derives from the connection between the chakra and the vowel. Moving up the musical scale at the same time, while eventually desirable, is not essential. If you cannot find C with your voice, simply intone the vowels with your focus on each chakra.

- Take a deep breath, and tone from the bottom chakra (root) to the top chakra (crown). Start with UH, then proceed through OO, OH, AH, EYE, AYE, EE. Do this in one breath if you are able.

- Breathe again, and reverse the process, toning from top (crown) to bottom (root). If this is too difficult at first, say each vowel separately, directing your attention to each chakra as you proceed.

- Once you've become more proficient, see if you can manage to tone in both directions in one breath.

- You can also start at the top, work to the bottom, and tone back to the top. Then stop, breathe normally, and see how you feel both physically and emotionally. Jonathan Goldman is a great proponent of this method and has written about it at length in his book *The Divine Name*.
- If you are chanting using the second table, place your focus on the root chakra, and use a short explosive breath to say *luhm, luhm, luhm*. It may feel like vocally beating a drum. Then move to the sacral chakra and chant *woom, woom, woom*. Proceed up the chakras to the third eye chakra. Hold OM on one long note. Similarly, you can hold NG for longer. Sustaining the note for OM and NG holds your focus in the third eye and the crown chakra allowing you to open to the divine.

Using either system, you don't have to visit all the chakras at once. You may decide to focus your chant on only one or two if you feel they need attention.

In addition to working with the chakras, each vowel has unique direct connections with the body.

UH is the sound of the root chakra and is associated with the gonads and ovaries and general vitality as this is where the kundalini energy originates at the base of the spine.

OO is concerned with the muscular system, the immune system, the adrenal glands, lower body circulation, and the natural functioning of the genital region, including the blood supply and tissues surrounding the area.

OH has a direct positive impact on the organs of the middle part of the body, including the liver, the pancreas, the stomach, the spleen, and the lower intestines. It may be helpful in shedding belly weight as it affects metabolism. It could also be useful to relieve constipation if used regularly.

AH is heart-strengthening. It carries the intention to improve blood flow and circulation. AH is sounded in the chest and affects the whole chest cavity, so toning this vowel would be useful in working with lung conditions such as a cough, shortness of breath, and asthma. It also stimulates the thymus and the immune system.

AYE is associated with the thyroid gland, metabolism, and body temperature. As it acts as the bridge between the heart and the mind, this vowel can help to balance emotions. Physically, it strengthens the soft membranes inside the vocal cord. Therefore, it is useful for singers or people who have to teach or give presentations where they will be speaking for some time beyond their natural volume.

EYE works with the pituitary gland and the medulla oblongata in the brain, which controls breathing, hearing, and taste. The pituitary gland regulates all the other glands in the body.

EE is at the crown of the head and is associated with the skeletal system as well as controls biological cycles and sleep patterns.

Vowels can be utilized to soothe and "open" parts of our body. To use this knowledge to maximum effect, prepare before you begin toning the chosen vowel by focusing on the part of the body it connects with. As you inhale, the power of the breath, or prana, will take energy to that location. As you exhale, sounding the vowel, you vibrate that area. So, you are using a triple power: intention, breath, and vibration. Intoning vowels in this way uses sonic resonance on spirit and body and resonates through the whole auric field (see page 13).

Turn it down!

At least once a week, give yourself a break and get away from it all. As we have seen, modern life is noisy and we weren't created to live this way. If you can't get out in the silence of nature, at least turn down the noise at home. Turn off the television. Take out the earbuds. Switch off the mobile. Perhaps invest in some noise canceling headphones for your journey to work if you take public transportation. Put on some ear defenders. The world is loud but you don't have to suffer from it.

Let It Out!

While unwanted noise is stressful, sometimes a great form of therapy is to make some noise.

- If you have a sense that you are angry or upset about something, take yourself to a safe space where you will not disturb others, and make some noise. Drum, stamp your feet, scream, or shout. Beating a cushion or pillow and letting rip vocally will release what is pent up inside, and the truth of what is behind your mood will probably come to you.

- I often go outside and tone OM as loudly as my human form will allow to waves, trees, rocks, and valleys, sending sonic vitamins of gratitude and love to all creation. What we give out returns to us threefold. The amount of breath required to execute this will energize you and release tension.

- If you can go outside to a remote location, you can fling open your arms and really let go. My yogi taught me that the arms are an extension of the heart. Tell the Universe your woes. Scream, yell, or do whatever else comes to you. Throwing a stone into water or the far distance is a good accompaniment to this. I find this technique is particularly useful when I am angry or disappointed in myself. Equally, it is a handy adjunct to the Serenity Prayer:

> *God, grant me the serenity to accept the things*
> *I cannot change,*
> *The courage to change the things I can,*
> *And the wisdom to know the difference.*

Let go, let rip, and let peace—that still, small voice of calm—fill the silence that follows.

Afterword

I HOPE YOU HAVE ENJOYED your journey through the many ways that intentional use of commonplace and sacred sound and vibration can be used therapeutically to balance and improve life spiritually, mentally, emotionally, and physically.

Sound soothes and guides us from the cradle to the grave. Whether it is a mother's lullaby, a loved one's words, music, chant, or sacred instruments, all are gifts to draw from when we need succor.

By reading this book, I hope you have found sonic vitamins to enrich your life's experience. I have included a resource section should you wish to research any of the vitamins in greater depth.

May the *Om* be with you!

Namaste.

ERICA LONGDON

Acknowledgments

WRITING A BOOK MAY SEEM as simple as committing thoughts, knowledge, and words to the page. However, like a performance on stage, so much support goes on backstage. This work would never have arrived in print without the initial encouragement, help, and guidance of Elaine Harrison, who champions and promotes Inner Traditions books here in the UK. Her help with my submission was vital. My heartfelt thanks also go to Leonie Bunch for all her support and advice in preparing the artwork. Words I can do; digital media is something I have yet to master. I am grateful to Jon Graham of Inner Traditions for believing in me and this book. My deep thanks go to Kayla Toher for nurturing me through the editing phase and all at Inner Traditions for their kind encouragement and patience as they guided me through the process of birthing this book.

Notes

INTRODUCTION. VIBRATION, THE FOUNDATION OF SOUND HEALING

1. "Professor Damien Coyle," Ulster University website, accessed April 16, 2020.
2. Larry Hardesty, "Computer System Transcribes Words Users 'Speak Silently'," MIT News, April 4, 2018.
3. Trevor English, "What Is the Schumann Resonance?" Interesting Engineering blog, October 25, 2019.
4. Jim Wilson, "Schumann Resonance," NASA website, May 28, 2013.
5. S. Danho, W. Schoellhorn, and M. Aclan, "Innovative Technical Implementation of the Schumann Resonances and Its Influence on Organisms and Biological Cells," *Materials Science and Engineering* 564 (2019).
6. "Global Coherence Research," HeartMath Institute website, accessed April 17, 2020.
7. Joe Dispenza, "What Does the Spike in the Schumann Resonance Mean?" Dr. Joe Dispenza's blog, accessed May 4, 2020.
8. "Music Therapist," The Health Careers website for the United Kingdom, accessed May 4, 2020.
9. David Hulse, *A Fork In the Road* (Bloomington, Ind.: AuthorHouse, 2009), 93.
10. John Beaulieu, *Human Tuning: Sound Healing with Tuning Forks* (New York: Biosonics, 2009), 56.

147

11. "A Brief History of Dr. Royal Raymond Rife," Royal Rife Machine website, accessed May 4, 2020.

VITAMIN B. BREATH, BOWLS

1. Gabriel Reilich (writer and director) and Jake Infusino (graphics), "The Breathing Earth: Climate Change Data Visualization," posted by GOOD Magazine, YouTube, November 24, 2015.
2. Sebastian Gendry, "Why Deep Breathing Matters, Activates the Vagus Nerve," Laughter Online University, accessed June 1, 2020; M. Rosas-Ballina and K. J. Tracey, "Cholinergic Control of Inflammation," *Journal of Internal Medicine* 265 no. 6 (2009): 663–79.
3. Olivia F. O'Leary et al., "The Vagus Nerve Modulates BDNF Expression and Neurogenesis in the Hippocampus" *Elsevier,* 28 no. 2 (February 2018): 307–16.
4. N. D. Theise and R. Harris, "Postmodern Biology: (Adult) (Stem) Cells Are Plastic, Stochastic, Complex, and Uncertain," *Handbook of Experimental Pharmacology* 174 (2006): 389–408.
5. Mitchell Gaynor, *Sounds of Healing: A Physician Reveals the Therapeutic Power of Sound, Voice, and Music* (New York: Broadway Books, 1999).
6. John Swain, "What Is the Science behind Quartz Crystals?" Boston.com, February 8, 2010.

VITAMIN C.
CYMATICS, CHAKRAS, CHANTING

1. Wikipedia, s.v. "Cymatics," accessed May 4, 2020.

VITAMIN D.
DRUMMING, DIDGERIDOO

1. Michael Drake, "Drumming the Hollow Bone," *Sacred Hoop Magazine* 78 (2012).
2. "The Benefits of Drumming," Project Resiliency website, accessed June 3, 2020.

3. Masatada Washi et al., "Recreational Music-Making Modulates Natural Killer Cell Activity, Cytokines, and Mood States in Corporate Employees," *Medical Science Monitor* 13 no. 2 (2007): 57–70.

4. Quoted by Linda Buch, "The Biological Benefits of Drumming," BioSync website, March 20, 2013.

5. Christiane Northrup, M.D., "10 Health Reasons to Start Drumming: The Health Benefits to Beating Your Own Drum," Dr. Northrup's website, March 21, 2016. Reprinted with permission.

6. Robert Eley, "The Potential Effects of the Didgeridoo as an Indigenous Intervention for Australian Aborigines: A Post Analysis," *Music and Medicine* 5 no. 2 (2013): 84–92; Robert Eley and Don Gorman, "Didgeridoo Playing and Singing to Support Asthma Management in Aboriginal Australians," *The Journal of Rural Health* (January 2010).

7. Milo A. Puhan et al., "Didgeridoo Playing as Alternative Treatment for Obstructive Sleep Apnoea Syndrome: Randomised Controlled Trial," *British Medical Journal* 332 (2006): 226.

VITAMIN F.
FREQUENCY, FORKS

1. J. Calvin Coffey and D. Peter O'Leary, "The Mesentery: Structure, Function, and Role in Disease," *The Lancet* 1 no. 3 (2016): 238–47.

2. For more information on ELF, see David S. Walonick, "Effects of 6-10 Hz ELF on Brain Waves," *Journal of Borderland Research* 46 no. 3–4 (1990). Available on the Borderlands Science website.

3. Grazyna Fosar and Franz Bludorf, "Scientist[s] Prove DNA Can Be Reprogrammed by Words and Frequencies," Dr. Joe Dispenza's blog, accessed May 4, 2020.

4. Denise Nolten, "Sound and the Influence of Sound on the Human Body," Gerrit Rietveld Academie thesis, 2012.

5. HeartMath Institute, *Science of the Heart: Exploring the Role of*

the Heart in Human Performance, Vol. 2. chapter 6. Available at the HeartMath website.

6. Simone Vitale, "432 Hz: A New Standard Pitch?" Sound of Golden Light website, accessed June 16, 2020.

7. John Beaulieu, "Tuning Fork, 432," Biosonics website, accessed June 16, 2020.

8. David Hulse, *A Fork in the Road* (Bloomington, Ind.: AuthorHouse, 2009).

VITAMIN L.
LISTENING, LAUGHTER

1. Andreas Bartels and Semir Ziki, "The Neural Correlates of Maternal and Romantic Love," *NeuroImage* 21 (2004): 1155–66; Andreas Bartels and Semir Ziki, "The Neural Basis of Romantic Love," *NeuroReport* 11 no. 17 (2000): 3829–34.

2. Kaitlin McLean, "Can Laughter Be Therapeutic?" *Yale Scientific Magazine,* May 12, 2011.

3. Thomas Flindt, *Laughter Yoga for Business and Pleasure* (Amazon Services, 2011).

VITAMIN M.
MANTRA, MUSIC, MMM HUMMING

1. F. H. Rauscher, G. L. Shaw, C. N. Ky, "Music and Spatial Task Performance," *Nature* 365 (1993): 611; J. S. Jenkins, "The Mozart Effect," *Journal of the Roayl Society of Medicine* 94 no. 4 (2001): 170–72.

2. Steven Morris, "Do You Know This Man? Mystery of the Silent, Talented Piano Player Who Lives for His Music." *The Guardian,* May 16, 2005.

3. Music & Memory, "Man in Nursing Home Reacts to Hearing Music from His Era," Youtube, November 18, 2011.

4. CBS News, "79-Year-Old with Dementia Remembers Song He Wrote Decades Ago, Plays It on Piano for Son," Youtube, June 26, 2019.

5. Peter Janata, "The Neural Architecture of Music-Evoked Autobiographical Memories," *Cerebral Cortex* 19 no. 11 (2009): 2579–94.

6. Kajmani (Kumud Ajmani), "Gayatri Mantra Word by Word Meaning," Glimpses of Divinity blog, January 25, 2018.

VITAMIN N.
NADA YOGA, NAME, NATURAL SOUNDS

1. Desh Kapoor, "Four Manifestations of Sound and Possible Ways to Communicate," Patheos website, August 30, 2009.

2. Baird Hersey, *The Practice of Nada Yoga: Meditation on the Inner Sacred Sound* (Rochester, Vt.: Inner Traditions, 2013).

VITAMIN O. *OM*

1. Elizabeth Howell, "Cosmic Microwave Background: Remnant of the Big Bang," Space.com, August 24, 2018.

2. "Did NASA Record OM Sound From The Sun? Here Is The Reality Check," Metrosaga website, January 4, 2020.

VITAMIN S. SILENCE

1. World Health Organization, *Burden of Disease from Environmental Noise. Quantification of Healthy Life Years Lost in Europe,* (2011).

2. P. D. Larsen and D. C. Galletly, "The Sound of Silence Is Music to the Heart," *Heart,* April 2006 92(4): 433–34.

3. Mitzi Baker, "Music Moves Brain to Pay Attention, Organize Events," Stanford News website, August 8, 2007.

4. Imke Kirste, Zeine Nicola, Golo Kronenberg, Tara L. Walker, Robert C. Liu, Gerd Kempermann, "Is Silence Golden? Effects of Auditory Stimuli and Their Absence on Adult Hippocampal Neurogenesis," *Brain Structure and Function* 220 (2015): 1221–28.

5. Rose Eveleth, "Earth's Quietest Place Will Drive You Crazy in 45 Minutes," *Smithsonian Magazine* website, December 17, 2013;

Jacopo Prisco, "Inside the World's Quietest Room," CNN website, March 28, 2018.

VITAMIN V.
VOICE, VOWELS, VOLUME

1. Don Campbell, *Healing Yourself with Your Own Voice* (Louisville, Colo.: Sounds True, 2015).
2. Melanie Braun, "Exploring the Efficacy of Vowel Intonations," *The Rose+Croix Journal,* 2005, 2: 12.
3. "Explore the Carvings," s.v. "Musical Cubes," Rosslyn Chapel website, accessed June 8, 2020.
4. Ellen Poliakov et al., "Effect of Background Noise on Food Perception," *Food Quality and Preference* 22 no. 1 (2011): 42–47.
5. United States Department of Labor, "Occupational Noise Exposure," USDL website, accessed June 8, 2020; Ellen Kerns and Elizabeth Masterson, "Workplace Noise: More than Just 'All Ears,'" CDC website, June 28, 2018.
6. Gisle Haakonsen and Tore Kleffelgård, "Noise Annoyance in Norway: 1999–2001," Statistics Norway website, March 13, 2003.
7. L. C. den Boer and A. Schoten, "Traffic Noise Reduction in Europe: Health Effects, Social Costs and Technical and Policy Options to Reduce Road and Rail Traffic Noise," Transport and Environment website, August 2007.

Resources

This is, by no means, an exhaustive list. It references the works by some of the teachers mentioned in this book and will lead to rich pastures of learning to deepen your practice.

BOOKS

Beaulieu, John. *Human Tuning: Sound Healing with Tuning Forks.* New York: BioSonic Enterprises, 2010.

Cousto, Hans. *The Cosmic Octave: Origin of Harmony.* Rev. ed. U.S.: LifeRhythm, 2000.

D'Angelo, James. *The Healing Power of the Human Voice: Mantras, Chants, and Seed Sounds for Health and Harmony.* Rochester, Vt.: Healing Arts Press, 2005.

Emoto, Masuro. *The Hidden Messages in Water.* Pocket Books; 2005.

Goldman, Jonathan and Andi. *The Humming Effect: Sound Healing for Health and Happiness.* Rochester, Vt.: Healing Arts Press, 2017.

Goldman, Jonathan. *The Divine Name: Invoke the Sacred Sound That Can Heal and Transform.* Rev. ed. Hay House, 2015.·

Hay, Louise. *You Can Heal Your Life.* Reprint, Hay House, 2008.

Hersey, Baird. *The Practice of Nada Yoga: Meditation on the Inner Sacred Sound.* Rochester, Vt.: Inner Traditions, 2013.

Hulse, David. *A Fork in the Road: An Inspiring Journey of How Ancient Solfeggio Frequencies Are Empowering Personal and Planetary Transformation.* Bloomington, Ind.: AuthorHouse, 2009.

Pearce, Stewart. *The Heart's Note: Sounding Love in Your Life from Your Heart's Secret Chamber.* Forres, Scotland: Findhorn Press, 2010.

Sturge, Lisa. *Laugh: Everyday Laughter Healing for Greater Happiness and Wellbeing.* Quadrille Publishing, 2017.

Swami Saradananda. *The Power of Breath: Yoga Breathing for Inner Balance, Health and Harmony.* London: Watkins Publishing, 2017.

Yogi Ashokananda. *The Power of Relaxation.* London: Watkins Publishing, 2015.

ONLINE RESOURCES & COURSES

If you would like to hear examples of some of the vitamins mentioned in this book, there is a free MP3 recording on my YouTube page. If you would like a unique MP3 crafted for you, there is also that option via my website Angelhandsheal. co.uk. I also offer in-person and remote sonic treatments.

To find a certified sound healing therapist in your area of the United Kingdom, visit the College of Sound Healing's website. In the United States, visit the Sound Healers Association website.

I recommend Tim Wheater's CD *Invisible Journeys,* produced by Gemini Sun Records in 2008. His website, timwheater .com, is also a valuable resource.

Gong master Mark Swan's website, www.gong-healing.com, provides information, details about workshops, and CDs to help you experience the power of the gong.

Visit www.biosonics.com to learn more about John Beaulieu and the information and products he offers, including CDs and tuning forks.

SuaraSoundHealing.com offers tuning fork training with Debbi Walker. The website also sells a variety of CDs and tuning forks as well as provides information.

Give a listen to Jonathan Goldman's recordings called *Chakra Chants* and *Chakra Chants 2.*

If you are interested in laughter yoga, visit the UnitedMind website if you live in the UK and the Laughter Yoga USA website if you live in the US.

Index